A SYSTE...
OF
CAUCASIAN YOGA

As Orally Received
By
Count Stefan Colonna Walewski

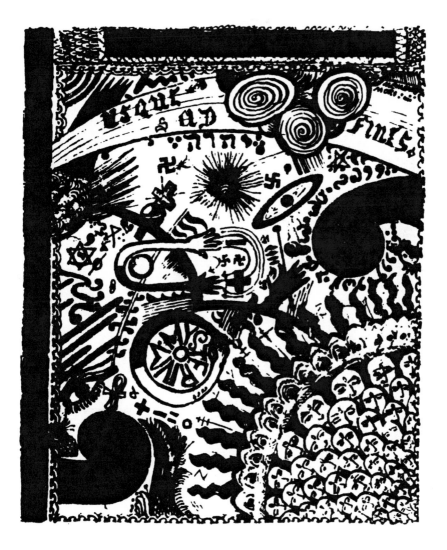

SYMBOLIC MONTAGE   S. C. WALEWSKI

KEY TO MASTERY

S

∴ I AM ON THIS EARTH.
TO RECLAIM THE EARTH.
TO TURN THE DESERTS INTO PARADISE
A PARADISE MUST SUITABLE
TO GOD AND HIS ASSOSIATES.
TO DWELL THEREIN. ∵

∵ ꝫꞇꞇꞇ ꞇꞷꝡ · ꞓꝺꞷ · ꞷꞇꞃꞷ ꞷꞇꞇ ∴

∴ YAT-HA-AHU-VAIRIO ∵

∴ THE WILL OF THE LORD IS
THE LAW OF RIGHTEOUSNESS ∵

— MASTERY —
YOU MUST.

INDEX.

CONTENTS

CONTENTS

CONTENTS

CONTENTS

CONTENTS

INTRODUCTION

IT WAS SAID 2000 YEARS AGO, THAT
THERE IS NOTHING HIDD THAT WOULD
NOT BE REVEALED.

In THIS KEY is GIVEN SIMPLIFIED,
CONDENSED, AND CORRECT MANNER
HOW TO MASTER, HOW To SOLVE EVERY
PROBLEM, ANSWER EVERY QUESTION,
in EVERY DEPARTAMENT OF LIFE, – IN
PHYSICAL, MENTAL, SPIRITUAL AND
PSYCHIC PLANES.

It is, THE KEY TO MEET EVERY SITUAION
BY APPLYING THE CONSCIUSLY DEVELOPED
    1) CAREFUL OBSERVATION
    2) CORRECT INTERPRETATION
& 3) PRACTICAL APLICATION.

To KNOW THYSELF – IS TO GO INSIDE
OF ONES ENTITY AND TO WATCH
STUDY AND APPLY.

INDICATOR OF ENTITY IS –
I – I AM, – SOUL
i THINK ;
i FEEL ;   }, ATTRIBUTES.
i WILL ;

INDICATOR OF THINKING, FEELING
AND WILLING IS THE BREATH.

8

A BEING IS BORN TO THIS WORLD, HAVING
AS BASIC RHYTM, - BREATH OF THE
MOTHER AT TIME OF THE CONCEPTION
THIS IS CALLED THE MOTHERS BREATH
AND WITHIN ITS VIBRATION ARE
HIDDEN THE DESTINY AND FATE OF
EVERY INDIVIDUAL.

PRODUCE THE CAUSES, AND THE EFFECTS
WILL FOLLOW.

STATE OF MASTERSHIP IS TO BE AT
ALL TIMES CONSCIUSLY IN POSITIVE
RECEPTIVE ATTITUDE, OPEN TO ALL
POSITIVE POWERS TO FLOW AND
EXPRESS THRU YOU.

AND TO DIRECT THEM IN THE
PROPER CHANNELS WHICH WILL
BE ILLUMINATED AND EXPRESS
GOOD THOUGHT, GOOD WORD, AND
GOOD WILL.

TITANIC POWER - GAYA LHAMA -
IS EVERYWHERE, AND ALWAYS
SEEKING ENTRANCE INTO HUMAN
BEING TO EXPRESS HERSELF THRU IT
TO BE RECEPTIVE TO THE HARMON-
IUS FLOW OF THIS POWER - IS TO
ESTABLISH MASTER RHYTM IN
THE HUMAN BEING AND RELINGON
THE MOTHERS IMPRESSION OF AD-
VERSE SOROUNDINGS. COINCIDENCES

9

AND INFLUENCES AT THE TIME OF CONCEPTION

BREATH IS LIFE.
FLOWING THRU THE NOSTRILS, BREATH
SHADES ITSELF THREE WAYS.
WHEN COMING THRU THE RIGHT NOSTRIL
IT IS CREATIVE ELECTRIC BREATH AND
IT IS FEEDING THE VASOMOTOR SYSTEM.
SO CALLED PINGALA. — NAME OF THIS
BREATH IS SUN BREATH. BREATH OF WARRIOR
READY TO FIGHT.

COMING THRU THE LEFT NOSTRIL
IT IS REGULATING AND MOTHERING
PRINCIPLE — MAGNETIC — IT IS FEEDING
THE SYMPATHETIC NERVOUS SYSTEM
SO CALLED — IDA — NAME OF THIS
BREATH IS — MOON BREATH.
BREATH OF THE SAGE READY TO ABSORB WISDOM.

COMING EVENLY THRU BOTH NOS-
TRILS IT IS BALANCING = PRESER-
VING OR DESTROYING. IT IS CALLED
       SHUSHUMNA BREATH

NORMALLY THE BREATH IS CHAN-
GING ABOUT EVERY HOUR —
SUN BREATH — NEUTRAL / SHUSHU-
MNA BREATH AND MOON BREATH
TWO POSTURES CREATE SUN
OR MOON BREATH IN 3 (THREE)
MINUTES. —
FOR THE SUN BREATH : LAY DOWN
ON THE LEFT SIDE, AND REST YOUR

10

HEAD ON THE LEFT HAND , THUMB OF
WHICH SHOULD BE TOUCHING THE CA
WITY UNDER LEFT EAR , REST OF THE
FINGERS COVERING THE FOREHEAD
  RIGHT ARM IS BENT UNDER STRAIGHT
ANGEL , WITH THE HAND RESTING ON
EARTH WITH THUMB POINTING IN THE
ASSYRIAN MANNER.
  HEEL OF THE RIGHT FOOT LAYS ON
THE KNEE JOINT OF THE LEFT LEG
HELD STRAITH. BY THIS POSTURE IT IS CHAN-
GED IN THREE MINUTES.

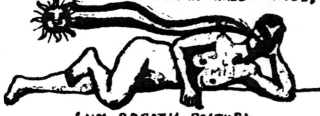

        SUN BREATH POSTURE
THE MOON BREATH IS THE SAME POSTURE
REVERSED +.
        ———————.·.———————

GAYA LHAMA - WHICH IS ENERGY
CONTAINED IN THE SPACE , HAS 4
(FOUR)STATES OF VIBRATION WHICH
CORRESPOND TO 4-(FOUR) COLORS
AND WHICH BEING ASSIMILATED
FROM THE AIR . HAVE CENTERS
IN THE HUMAN BODY AND VIVFY
THEM. -
THOSE VIBRATIONS ARE CORRESPON-
DING TO FOURFOLD FUNCTIONS OF
HUMAN ENTITY, AND ARE DEVELO
PING THEM.
                11

DEVELOPEMENT OF HUMAN ENTITY IS
FOURFOLD:—

1) PHYSICAL   3) SPIRITUAL
2) MENTAL   4) PSYCHIC.

COLORS CORRESPONDING TO THOSE
FUNCTIONS ARE.:—
1) RED -FOR THE PHYSICAL.
2) YELLOW -FOR THE MENTAL.
3) BLUE -FOR THE SPIRITUAL.
4) WHITE -FOR THE PSYCHIC.
PARTS OF THE BODY HOLDING THOSE VIB-
RATIONS ARE.

1) LOWER STOMACH; SEX; & BACK OF THE HEAD
   RED — PHYSICAL.∴

2) UPPER CHEST; & FOREHEAD — YELLOW —
   —MENTAL [INTELLECT].∴

3) SOLAR PLEXUS [ABDOMEN] & TOP OF THE
   HEAD — SPIRITUAL [VITIC ENERGY] BLUE:

4) ARMS, HANDS; LEGS, FEET & FACE —
   —WHITE — PSYCHIC.∴ [FOR WHITE RACE].∴

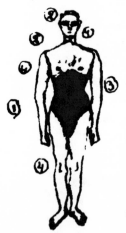 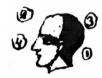

HUMAN BODY THRU CONSCIOUS
USE OF WILL BRETHS IN THE
COLOR VIBRATION, AND
AT EXHALATION CHARGES
PARTS AND CENTERS.
WHEN IT IS DONE IN THIS
WILLFUL AND. CONSCIOUS
MANNER IT IS BASIC
PART OF MASTER EXERCIZE

12

MASTER ARCANES, GREATER MYSTE
RIES.   GENERAL POINTS

A MASTER BREATH is 7 SECONDS IN-
HALATION — 7 SEC. EXHALATION AND 1
SECOND STOP OR HOLD AT EACH END/16
.THE MASTER RHYTM IS 7 SECONDS.
THIS CORRESPOND TO THE RHYTM OF
THE HEART CENTER (ESOTERIC) OF THE
EARTH .— + (PLUS) (WITH THE PAUSE OF
1 SECOND) (+).

THE EYES ARE TO BE RELAXED AS TO
MUSCULAR STRUCTURE .AND MUST NOT
BE FULLY CHARGED WITH POWER FROM
WITHIN . IN MASTER ESERCISES THE EYES
MUST PLAY. [HANG] ON THE SUN , MOON.
BEFORE THEY CROSS THE MERIDIAN , STAR
LIGHT, OR A SPOT .

SPOT USED AS EXERCIZE POINT MUST BE
ON WHITE BACKGROUND AND CAN BE FOR
GENERAL PURPOZES BLACK ON WHICH
THE CHARGING COLORS SHOULD BE IMA-
GINED MENTALLY . SIZE HAVE TO BE
ABOUT LIKE 1 CENT.

THE LIGHT OR SHINE , RADIATION AND
EMANATION OR REFLECTION OF EACH
OF HEAVENLY BODIES IS CALLED —
SUN SHINE ; MOON SHINE , STAR SHINE
ET.C. .˙.
EYES ABSORB OR EMANATE AMONG
OTHERS THE N OR LOVE RAYS, AND
THAT WHY THEY ARE THE INDEX OF
THE SOUL — SENDING OUT . LOVE,
WILL AND THOUGHT.
MASTER THOUGHT IS THE OPPO-
SITE OF SLAVE THOUGHT AS IS

13

MASTER WILL AND FEELING, AND
WE MUST MSTER OUR THOUGHT,
OUR WILL, AND OUR FEELINGS. - BY
RELAXATION IN POSITIVE ATTITUDE;
RELAXED BODY, BUT ALERT AND WATCH
FUL THOUGT, WILL AND FEELING, SO
WE ATTAIN TO RADIO-AUDIO RECEPTION
AND TRANSMISSION AT ONE AND THE
SAME TIME. AS MASTERS WE ARE
THE TRANSMITTER AND THE RE-
CEIVER: THE ECLESIS, SYNTHESIS
AND ANALYSIS:- THE FILLER,
THINKER AND WILLER.

HERTZ WAVES ARE THOUGHT
WAVES OF THE GEOID ENTITY
THE EARTH SOUL — ARMAITI —
WHOSE AURA WE BLEND WITH
OUR OWN IN THE SIXTH (6th)
MASTER ARCANE. EXERCISE :.

WHEN CONCENTRATING, MEDITATING
RECEVING OR SENDING ENERGY, THOUGB
MASTER ALWAYS FACES DIRECTION IN
WHICH SUN IS SITUATED AT GIVEN
MOMENT. EAST IN THE MORNING,
SOUTH AT NOON, WEST AT SUNSET,
AND NORTH AT MIDNIGHT, UNLESS
THERE IS A SPECIAL NEED OF MOON
POWER FOR ASTRAL, OR SPECIFIC
POWERS OF DIFFERENT PLANETS OR
STARS.- ACCORDING TO THEIR MAGICAL
PROPERTIES.

I -FIRST MASTER ARCANE. |EXERCISE

SIT ON A CHAIR - SPINE ERECT, NECK
STRAIGHT, HEAD UP, CHIN IN, EYES
LEVEL- FIXED ON SUN, OR SPOT WHICH
SHOULD BE ON THE LEVEL WITH THE
EYES AND ABOUT FROM THREE (3) to
SEVEN FEET AWAY ON A VERTICAL
WALL OR STAND.—REMEMBER LEVELS
OR HORISONTALS, VERTICALS OR PERPEN-
DICULARS, AND DIAGONALS, ANGLES,
STANDICULARS.

NOTE WHETER IN SUN OR MOON
BREATH. SUN - RIGHT NOSTRIL IS
HEATING AND ELECTRICAL. MOON
- LEFT NOSTRIL is COOLING AND
MAGNETIC..

RELAX ALL THE MUSCLES, BUT THOSE
THAT KEEP BACK AND NECK STRAIG
HT. REST THE HANDS WITH FINGERS
SLIGHTLY SEPARATES FORMING Vs
CN THIGHS, INDEX FINGERS AT KNEE
POINT AND THUMBS' CIRCLING TO THE
INSIDE OF TH KNEES.

HEELS FROM (3) THREE TO SIX (6) IN-
CHES APART FEET OPENED TO FORM
V, AND ALSO SHINS AND THIGS.
LIFE ATTRACTS LIFE, SYMBOL V HAS
CONCENTRATING POWER, AND SOUNDS V
AND (F) AND (PH) HAVE DIRECT MANTRIC
INVOKING) POWER TO ATTRACT,
INCREASE AND PROLONG.

15

KEEP YOUR THOUGHT FIXED ON GAYA-
LHAMA —[GA-EL-LHA-MAH] THE CEN-
TRALIZING PRINCIPLE OF LIFE, WHI.
CH IS ONLY APPROPRIATED BY LOVING
OF (AND SO ATTRACTING) THINKING
OF AND WILLING IT. THIS ACT BY
THOSE THREE POWERS FIXES THIS
ENERGY IN THE PHYSICAL, INTELL-
ECTUAL, SPIRITUAL AND PSYCHIC
EQUATION. ∴

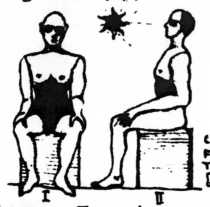

CORRECT POSTURE
FOR THE FIRST MAS
TER ARCANE
[EXERCIZE] ∴

I·FRONT ; II PROFILE ; III HAND ∴
[THE POSTURE IS THE SAME IN EGYPTIAN
RITUAL — ONLY IN EXOTERIC DOCTRINE IT
WAS SHOWN WITH LIMBS BROUGHT TO-
GETER, WITHOUT SHOWING THE STATE
OF RELAXATION PARTAINING TO
ESOTERIC DOCTRINE]. ‐
∴ HAVING THE POSTURE PROPERLY
TAKEN, BREATH IN FOR SEVEN (7)
SECONDS GAYA LHAMA — OF RED COLOU
EXPANDING ABDOMEN ; PAUSE ONE
SECOND ; THAN EXHALE THE BREATH

(AIR) FOR SEVEN (7) SECONDS, AT THE SAME TIME BY THOUGHT AND WILLING COLOUR - LOWER STOMACH, SEX AND BACK OF THE HEAD - RED PAUSE ONE SECOND, AND REPEAT SAME BREATH ON THE SAME COLOUR TWICE, TO MAKE THREE BREATHS ON RED COLOUR .∴

∴ THEN AFTER LAST PAUSE OF ONE SECOND PROCEED TO TAKE BREATH EXPANDING ONLY CHEST - (MENTAL) ON YELLOW COLOUR ; PAUSE 1 SECOND EXHALE FOR SEVEN SECONDS, FIXING BY THOUGHT AND WILLING YELLOW COLOR — CHEST AND FOREHEAD, PAUSE ONE SECOND AND REPEAT TO MAKE THREE BREATHS ON YELLOW COLOUR ∴

∴ AFTER LAST PAUSE OF ONE SECOND PROCEED TO TAKE BREATH EXPANDING CHEST AND UPPER ABDOMEN — ON BLUE (SPIRITUAL) COLOUR ; PAUSE ONE SECOND, EXHALE FOR SEVEN SECONDS, FIXING BY THOUGHT AND WILLING BLUE COLOUR — SOLAR PLEXUS [ABDOMEN. (DIAPHRAGM)], PAUSE ONE SECOND AND REPEAT TO MAKE THREE BREATHS ON BLUE COLOUR .∴

∴ AFTER LAST PAUSE OF ONE SECOND PROCEED TO TAKE BREATH EXPANDING LIKE IN RED BREATH - CHEST, DIAPHRAGM AND ABDOMEN — ON WHITE COLOUR .

17

PAUSE ONE SECOND, EXHALE FOR SEVEN
SECONDS - FIXING BY THOUGHT AND
WILLING WHITE COLOUR - ARMS, HANDS
LEGS, FEET AND FACE. PAUSE ONE SE-
COND AND REPEAT SAME BREATH TO
MAKE THREE BREATHS ON WHITE COLOUR::
∴ FULL BREATH WILL CONSIST OF
ONE INHALATION OF SEVEN - 7 SECONDS
ONE PAUSE OF ONE ----- — 1 SECOND
ONE EXHALATION OF SEVEN — 7 SECONDS
ONE PAUSE OF ONE --- — 1 SECOND

SUM ONE BREATH SIXTEEN   16 SECONDS
∴ TAKING THREE BREATHS FOR
EVERY DEVELOPEMENT SUM 16:
: 3 BREATHS ON RED (PHYSICAL)¹⁶ˢᵉᵃ 48 SEC
3 BREATHS ON YELLOW (MENTAL)   48 SEC.
3 BREATHS ON BLUE (SPIRITUAL)   48 SEC
3 BREATHS ON WHITE (PSYCHIC)   48. SE.

12 BREATHS   192 SEC.

ONE HUNDRED AND NINETY TWO SE-
CONDS , - OR THREE MINUTES AND
TWELVE SECONDS. 3'12".
WHICH COMPRISES A FULL 1ˢᵗ
MASTER EXERCIZE OF TWELVE
BREATHS IN 3 MINUTES AND
12 SECONDS. ∴
NOTE: BEFORE STARTING ON ANY
OF THE MASTER ARCANES (EXERCISES)
FIRST EXHALE ALL BREATH USING

18

MUSCLES OF THE ABDOMINAL
DIAPHRAGMATIC AND CHEST SECTIONS
TO EXPEL ALL RESIDUAL AIR.
∴. FIRST MASTER ARCANE, AWAKE-
NS FORCES OF THE UNIVERSE, GETS
IN TOUCH WITH THE HIGHER POWE-
RS, ESTABLISHES THE MASTER RHYTM
AND DEVELOPES CLAIRVOYANCE∴

II. SECOND MASTER ARCANE [EXERCISE]

STAND ERECT - SPINE AND NECK STRAIGHT
HANDS AT SIDES. RIGHT OR LEFT FOOT
FORWARD.(ACCORDING TO THE BREATH
YOU ARE IN) ABOUT 8 EIGHT INCHES.
EYES LEVEL FIXED LIKE IN FIRST EXER-
CISE.
EXHALE ALL BREATH USING MUSCLES OF
THE ABDOMINAL DIAFRAGMATIC AND
CHEST SECTIONS TO EXPEL ALL RESI-
DUAL AIR.∴
   INHALE FOR SEVEN (7) SECONDS
RISING ON TOES AND CLENCHING
HANDS TIGHTLY AS IF TO HOLD ON
TO LIFE PRINCIPLE IN THE AIR,
IMAGINE RED [GAYA-LHAMA]. PHYSICAL-
EXPANDING ABDOMEN, PAUSE ONE
SECOND (1); EXHALE SEVEN SECONDS
LOWERING TO THE FLOOR JUST TOUCHING
HEELS, AND UNCLENCHING HANDS
[DURING EXHALATION], CHARGING
LOWER ABDOMEN AND BACK OF THE
HEAD WITH RED. PAUSE ONE
19

SECOND, THEN BEGIN AGAIN TWO (2)
MORE BREATHS ON RED [PHYSICAL]
FOLLOW WITH THREE (3) BREATHS
ON YELLOW [INTELLECTUAL] ; THREE
(3) BREATHS ON BLUE (SPIRITUAL),
AND THREE (3) BREATHS ON WHITE
(PSYCHIC) USING SAME EXPANSIONS
AS DESCRIBED IN FIRST MASTER
ARCANE. ".'
TWELVE (12) BREATHS WILL CON-
STITUTE SECOND MASTER ARCA-
NE ".' 3 MINUTES 12 SECONDS ".'

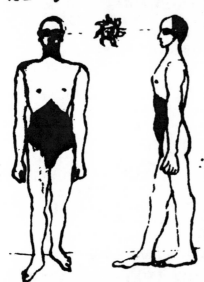

ILLUSTRATION
SHOWS POSTURE
FIRST, OF THE.
SECOND EXERCISE.
SECOND POSTURE
WILL BE ON RISED
TOES.
[THE SAME POSTU
RE IS IN EGYPTIAN
RITUAL] ".'
".WHICH FOOT TO
PUT FORWARD
DEPENDS ON THE
BREATH.
IN SUN BREATH
RIGHT FOOT, IN
MOON — THE
LEFT. .'

SECOND MASTER ARCANE TEACHES US
HOW TO FACE FRIENDS AND ENEMIES,
HOW TO DEFEND AND AGRESS. IT DEVE-
LOPES CLAIRAUDIENCE AND HAR-

20

MONY.

∴ NOTE: BATHE FEET WITH SOAP AND WATER, OR USE ALCOHOL RUB. COLD WATER IS USED FOR MAGNETIC SHOCK AND HOT FOR ELECTRIC [AMPERAGE].

WADING IN RIVERS, BROOKS OR EVEN TUB, DEWY GRASS OR SEA, IS MAGNETIC. WALKING ON DUSTY ROADS, SAND EARTH. IS ELECTRIC.∴

DRY FEET WELL, AND RUB THEM WELL WITH HANDS, THAN USE SOME OIL — [SWEET ALMOND OIL], COCONOUT OR COCOA BUTTER, CRUDE OIL AND KEROSENE ARE GOOD ALSO. NEWER USE ANIMALOIDS OTHER THAN LANOLIN [FROM SHEEP'S WOOL] OR BUTTER.∴

TAKE SPECIAL CARE. TO KEEP GREAT TOE IN GOOD CONDITION, MASAGE IT THOROUGHLY AND STRETCH AND PULL WITH HANDS TO. PREVENT NUMBNESS FROM SETTING IN IT. AND KEEP IT RESPONSIVE AND ALIVE.

GREAT TOE IS CONNECTED WITH HEARING [AUDITORY NERVE] AND COORDINATES HARMONY, AND RHYTM IN THE BODY.

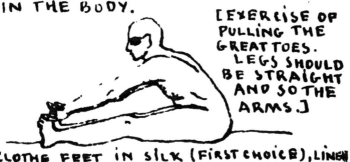

[EXERCISE OF PULLING THE GREAT TOES.
LEGS SHOULD BE STRAIGHT AND SO THE ARMS.]

CLOTHE FEET IN SILK (FIRST CHOICE), LINEN

OR WOOL, OR COTTON AND DRAW STO-
CKING OR SOCKS ON OVER CLOTH.
∴ CHANGE FOOT CLOTHS WHENEVER
FEET ARE MOIST AND COLD, THIS
PREVENTS COLDS, COUGHS, AND
AFFECTIONS OF EARS, EYES AND TH-
ROAT, AS WELL AS MANY RHEUMATIC
CONDITION, TO A GREAT EXTENT.

III THIRD MASTER ARCANE [EXERCISE]
SIT ON A CHAIR - SPINE ERECT NECK
STRAIGHT, HEAD UP - AS IN FIRST MASTER
ARCANE [EXERCISE]. HAVE ONE SPOT
FIXED LEVEL WITH THE EYES [OR
USE SUN, MOON E.T.C.] AND THE OTHER
THREE (3) TO FOUR (4) FEET DISTANT
ON THE EARTH (FLAT ON IT) OR ON THE
FLOOR. NOTE WHETHER IN THE SUN
OR MOON BREATH.
RELAX ALL THE MUSCLES, BUT THOSE THAT
∴ KEEP BACK AND NECK STRAIGHT. REST
THE HANDS WITH FINGERS SLIGHTLY
SEPARATED - FORMING V'S ON THIGHS;
INDEX FINGERS AT KNEE POINT AND THUMB
ENCIRCLING TOWARD INSIDE OF THE KNEES,
∴ HEELS FROM THREE TO SIX INCHES, APART
FEET OPEN TO FORM V; AND ALSO SHINS
AND THIGHS. ∴ HAVING THE POSTURE PRO-
PERLY TAKEN (EXHALE ALL AIR) START RHYTMICALLY BEND
FORWARD, KEEPING SPINE AND NECK
IN LINE, SHIFT EYES TO THE GROUND
(FLOOR) SPOT; INHALING FOR SEVEN

SECONDS, EXPANDING ABDOMEN, AND
TAKING IN RED GAYA-LHAMA (PHYSICAL
WHILE INHALING, CONCENTRATE ON
LIFE PRINCIPLE ACKNOWLEDGING AND MENTALLY SAY:
:" __BREATH__ IS LIFE ", HOLD ONE (1)
SECOND WHEN RIBS TOUCH THIGHS
AND MENTALLY SAY :" BREATH __IS__
LIFE ":, FIXING PRINCIPLE OF LIFE
BY AFFIRMING ;.. EXHALE FOR SEVEN
(7) SECONDS, RISING ERECT TO ORIGI-
NAL STARTING POSTURE, CHARGING
LOWER ABDOMEN AND BACK OF THE
HEAD - RED - MENTALLY SAYING
:" BREATH IS __LIFE__ " REALIZING AND
AFFIXING PRINCIPLE OF LIFE.
WHEN EXHALING AND RISING SHIFT
EYES TO HORIZONTAL SPOT OR
CENTER,.." THEN AFTER PAUSE FOR
ONE (1) SECOND BEGIN AGAIN TWO
MORE BREATHS ON RED (PHYSICAL)
FOLLOW WITH THREE BREATHS ON
YELLOW (INTELLECTUAL); PROCEED
WTH THREE BREATHS ON BLUE
(SPIRITUAL) AND CLOSE WITH THREE
BREATHS ON WHITE (PSYCHIC),
USING EXPANSIONS AS DESCRIBED
IN FIRST MASTER ARCANE. TWELVE
BREATHS - ONE MASTER EXERCIZE,
TIME THREE MINUTES TWELVE SE-
CONDS..."
GENERAL NOTE: WITH ALL THE MASTER
ARCANES, ALWAYS NOTE IN WHAT

BREATH YOU ARE , WHEN BENNING EXER-
CISES (AND WATCH. TO HAVE EVEN
NUMBER OF EXERCISES ON EVERY
BREATH . iE. IF IN THE MORNING YOU
WERE DOING EXERCISES WHILE IN SUN
(RIGHT NOSTRIL) BREATH , MAKE THE
EXERCISES IN THE AFTERNOON OR
WHEN MAKING THEM NEXT TIME
PAY ATTENTION TO BE IN THE MOON
(LEFT NOSTRIL) BREATH ...

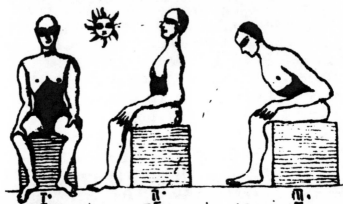

I. FRONT VIEW OF III EXERCIZE [BEGINNING THE
   INHALATION AND END OF EXHALATION.
II SAME AS ABOVE (PROFILE) . " " " "
III PROFILE VIEW AT THE END OF INHALATION
   AND BEGINNING EXHALATION.
.'. THOUGHT FIXED ON GAYALHAMA [GA-EL-
-LHA-MA] , EYES ON HORIZONTAL SPOT,
AND ON EARTH (FLOOR) SPOT: THIS THIRD
MASTER ARCANE DEVELOPES GOOD
TASTE AND JUDGEMENT OF DISTANCE
HOLDING THE CONSTANT ATTRACTION
OF GREAT CENTRALISING PRINCIPLE
2 I AM BREATHING LIFE IN ON

24

MY BREATH — AND FORMING A FIELD
OF MAGNETIC FORCE AROUND ME,
MY MAGNETIC FIELD OR AURA :.'"

IV FOURTH MASTER ARCANE [EXERCISE]
STAND ERECT — SPINE AND NECK STRA-
IGHT, FEET EIGHTHEN TO TWENTY FOUR
INCHES APART, RISE HAND ABOVE EYES
(ABOUT 18" FROM THE EYES) PALM TOWARD
YOU, KEEP EYES ON SPOT (LEVEL WITH
EYES), SUN OR MOON. THOUGHT AND
WILL FIXED ON GA-EL-LHA-MAH .
NOTE IN WHAT BREATH YOU ARE .
EXHALE ALL RESIDUAL AIR FROM THE
LUNGS USING MUSCLES OF THE ABDOMI-
NAL DIAPHRAGMATIC AND CHEST SECTIONS.
.'. NOW, ROTATE ARM RAPIDLY, ONE
REVOLUTION A SECOND, [NOTE : EXERCIE
SHOULD B ALWAYS STARTED WITH THE ARM
ON THE SIDE IN WHICH BREATH I- FLO-
WING, AND ROTATION SHOULD BE MADE
TOWARD THE BODY, CUTTING OF VISION
EVERY CIRCLE.). BREATH IN RED GA-
YALHAMA FOR SEVEN SECOND MAKIN
SEVEN CIRCLES WITH ARM (USING
MOMENTUM); AFTER INHALATION
AND ROTATION LET THE ARM DROP
RELAXED (LIMP) TO THE SIDE, USING
TIME ONE SECOND PAUSE . RISE SAME
HAND AND ARM AGAIN AND EXHALING
FOR SEVEN SECONDS AND ROTATING
SEVEN TIMES — AT THE SAME TIME
CHANGE LOWER ABDOMEN AND BACK

OF THE HEAD WITH RED -. PHYSICAL.
AT THE END OF EXHALATION ~~OR~~ LET
THE ARM DROP AT ITS OWN MOMEN-
TUM TOTHE SIDE .˙.
PAUSE ONE SECOND ˙.
.˙. INHALING NOW RAISE ARM FULL
LENGTH OVER SHOULDER CLENCHING
HAND, TIME SEVEN SECONDS. [BREATH
-RED-PHYSICAL]. TENSE AND SLIGHTLY
VIBRATE CLENCHED HAND. RAPIDLY
BEND AND ~~STRIKE~~ THE EARTH IN
FRONT OF THE FEET WITH FIST, LET-
TING GO THE MOMENT YOU STRIKE,
OF BREATH AND GRIP .˙.
RAISE BODY ERECT THROWING THE
HAND AND ARM UP BACK, AND DOWN
THE SIDE WITH ROUND GRACEFUL MO-
TION, MAKING TIME SEVEN SE-
CONDS MOTION AND EXHALATION,
CHARGING RED TO THE LOWER
ABDOMEN AND BACK OF THE HEAD .˙.
.˙. PAUSE ONE SECOND ˙.
REPEAT BOTH PARTS OF EXERCISE
ON THE SAME COLOR (RED) IN OTHER
ARM .˙. IN THIS MASTER ARCANE
YOU TAKE FOUR BREATHS ON A COLOUR
(TWO ON THE BREATH AND TWO COMPLI-
MENTORY.) .˙. MAKING IN ALL SIX-
TEEN BREATHS (16), 4 ON RED -PHY-
SICAL, FOUR (4) ON YELLOW -MENTAL
FOUR ON BLUE -SPIRITUAL, AND
FOUR ON WHITE -PSYCHIC.

26

SO THE FOURTH MASTER ARCANE (EXER-
CISE IN ITS EVERY DEVELOPEMENT
COLOR - CONSISTS OF TWO PARTS.

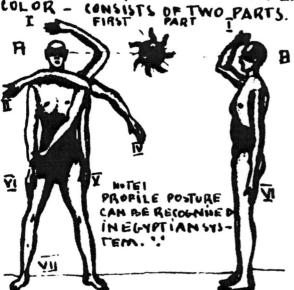

FIRST PART I

NOTE!
PROFILE POSTURE
CAN BE RECOGNIZED
IN EGYPTIAN SYS-
TEM. ∴

ABOVE ILLUSTRATION SHOWS FIRST PART OF POSTURE
OF THE FOURT MASTER ARCANE. IV EXERCISE
A - FRONT VIEW ; B - PROFILE ∴
A - I - BEGINNING POSTURE POSITION B - I
A - I - II - III - IV - I ; CIRCLE DESCRIBED
IN ROTATING ARM.
A - IV - V - ARM DROPING TO THE SIDE
AFTE SEVEN ROTATIONS.
A - VI - ARM AND HAND NOT IN USE.
(RELAXED). ∴
A - VII - FEET SPREAD. ∴
NOTE: AFTER GOING THROUGH THE FIRST
PART OF EXERCISE (ONE BREATH) PROCEED
WITHOUT ⌐BUT REGULAR INTERMIDIATE

27

ONE SECOND (1s.)] STOP INTO THE SECOND
PART OF THE EXERCISE. SO AS TO KEEP
EXERCISE AS A WHOLE. SO AS TO KEEP
SECOND PART :-

A

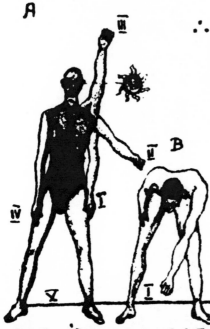

∴ PROFILE IS NOT
DRAWN BECAUSE
THE FRONT VIEW
CLEARLY EXPRES-
SES — THE EXERCISE

THIS PART ALWAYS
BEGINS WITH THE
ARM AND HAND
FROM THE SIDE
IN WHICH THE
BREATH IS FLOWING
AND THAN ON
THE OTHER SIDE.

FRONT VIEW OF THE SECOND. PART OF
THE FOURTH ARCANE (EXERCISE):
A-I- BEGINNING , A-II T A-III - INHALING
AND LIFTING THE ARM — GRADUALLY
TENSING THE GRIP.
FIGURE B. : B-I- DURING ONE (1)
SECOND PAUSE IN BREATH BENDING
FROM THE POSITION IN. A-III THROGH
POSITION B-I- TO STRIKE THE EARTH
(AT THE SAME TIME RELEASING THE
BREATH AND GRIP, THAN WHILE

28

EXHALING STRAIGHTEN UP AND THROUGH
POSITION B-I, BUT WIT GRIP RELAXED
BRING ARM TO POSITION A-III, THAN
A-II- THAN FINALLY A-I.-TO START
AFTER ONE SECOND (I) PAUSE AGAIN
ON THE OTHER ARM AND HAND A-IV..
  THIS FOURTH MASTER ARCANE (EXER-
-CISE) IS DEVELOPING THE COMMANDING
WILL- AND ELECTRICITY, STORING
IT IN GANGLIAS OF THE BODY, READY
TO USE. .:

V FIFTH MASTER ARCANE [EXER CISE].:. STAND ERECT, SPINE AND NECK

STRAIGHT, FEET THRE TO SIX INCHES APART,
SLIGHTLY BENT IN THE KNEES. RELAX ALL
MUSCLES. NOTICE THE BREATH YOU ARE
IN - SUN OR MOON. KEEP EYES ON SUN
MOON OR THE SPOT. THOUGHT AND WILL
FIXED ON GA-EL-LHA-MAH. .:.
.:. RAISE HANDS AND ARMS FROM THE
BACK OVER HEAD TO FRONT, LEVEL
WITH SHOULDERS.:
„FLOAT„ ARMS ON AIR AS IF ABOUT TO
FLY. HANDS LIMP FROM THE WRIST.:
EXHALE ALL RESIDUAL AIR FROM THE
LUNGS, USING MUSCLES OF THE AB-
DOMINAL DIAPHRAGMATIC AND CHEST
SECTIONS, AND FIX YOUR THOUGHT
ON COLOR RED-PHYSICAL .:.

29

∴ INHALE FOR SEVEN SECONDS AND TEN-
SE ARM MUSCLES. TO WRIST ONLY, LEA-
VING THEM LIMP, EXPANDING FOR PHY-
SICAL-RED COLOUR LOWER ABDOMEN.
PAUSE ONE SECOND. ∴

EXHALE FOR SEVEN SECONDS, RELAXING
AND FOLDING ARMS ON BREAST, RIGHT
HAND ON RIGHT BREAST, LEFT HAND
ON LEFT BREAST, AT THE SAME TIME
CHARGING LOWER ABDOMEN AND
BACK OF THE HEAD WITH RED COLOUR
PHYSICAL. DO IT ON EVERY COLOUR.

RED-PHYSICAL ; YELLOW-MENTAL
BLUE-SPIRITUAL AND WHITE-PSY-
CHIC. THREE TIMES. (12 BREATHS.)

NOTE: LEGS HAVE TO BE
SLIGHTLY BENT IN THE
KNEES.

∴ IN PROFILE
EXERCISE IS SHOWN
WITH MOTION OF ONE
ARM ONLY ∴

30

∴ NOW AGAIN EXTEND AND CIRCLE
HANDS ON LEVEL OF SHOULDERS TO
SIDES, TENSING MUSCLES OF ARMS
(HANDS LIMP), FOLD AND AXTEND
AGAIN AT SIDES E.T.C. ON EVERY
COLOUR (THREE TIMES.)
THEN AT THE LAST BREATH, RETURN
TO THE FRONT BUT SWING HANDS UP
FINGERS TOWARD EACH OTHER BUT
NOT TOUCHING, NOW DROP AND
EXHALE THROUGH MOUTH QUICKLY
SAYING HÂ AS IN HA HA, BUT
LONG SIGH LIKE BREATH, SWINGING
ARMS LIMP AS THE LESSION GOES∷
   NOW TO EXPLAIN CORRECTLY,
ON EVERY COLOR (PHYSICAL, MENTAL
SPIRITUAL AND PSYCHIE, THERE
ARE THREE BREATHS — TWO WITH
HANDS IN FRONT AND ONE WITH
HANDS ON THE SIDES, ALL TOGE-
THER 12 TWELVE BREATHS
   THIS FIFTH MASTER ARCANE IS
ONE WHICH GIVES CONTROL OVER
ATTRACTION OF THE EARTH, (WEIGHT)
ENABLING TO RAISE IN THE AIR,
FLY, AND WALK ON WATER.∴

VI MASTER ARCANE [EXERCISE]

∴ 1) STAND ERECT (3) THREE FEET
AWAY FROM THE BACK OF A CHAIR WITH
STRAIGHT ROUND POLES IN THE BACK
(UPRIGHT, VERTICAL), OR INSTEAD OF
A CHAIR USE TWO STAFFS OF BAMBOO
OR OTHER MATERIAL. —

2) HOLDING THE UPRIGHT POLES, KNEEL
CLOSE TO THEM, (OR TO THE CHAIR) BY
BALANCING ON BALLS OF THE FEET,
AND BENDING BACK TO MAINTAIN
BALANCE AS YOU KNEEL. [RELAX]
AFTER KNEELING.

3) HOLD BACK OF THE CHAIR (OR THE POLES),
GENTLY, AND EMPTY LUNGS. — THORO-
GHLY, BUT GENTLY AND EASILY.

4) INHALE FOR SEVEN (7) SECONDS
AND TIGHTEN GRIP AS YOU INHALE.

5) KEEP EYES FOCUSED ON THE SPOT -
LEVEL WITH THEM ON THE WALL OR
SCREEN WITHOUT STRAINING OR STA-
RING, SHIFT EYES AROUND THE "SPOT"
CIRCUMFERENCE, SIZE OF A PENNY.

⊕ [EXPLAINING LINE OF DECLINATION.
NECK AND SPINE STRAIGHT, BODY ERECT
CHIN IN - ALL MUSCLES RELAXED. FEET
STRAIGHT OR RIGHT ANGLE, OR HEELS

32

OUT ⬚ OR (FIRST) EXCITATION OF
∧ ∧,

FUNCTIONS BY RAPID PANTING —THEN
(SECOND) —BREATHE ALL AIR OUT USING
MUSCLES OF TRUNK, ABDOMEN AND
DIAPHRAGM TO DRIVE RESIDUAL AIR
CUT, AS MUCH AS POSSIBLE.
BREATH MAY BE SNIFFED, SOBBED,
OR WAVED IN, BUT- SIGHED OUT.—]
6) ▆▆▆▆▆▆▆▆▆▆▆▆▆ NOW AFTER
INHALING HOLD BREATH FOR SEVEN
(1) SECONDS, THIS IS CALLED KUMBHAKA
(IN HINDOO) IN YOGAH, TO HOLD OR MASTER
THE BREATH. [WHILE HOLDING BREATH EXERT A
GENTLE PRESSURE AGAINST THE DIAPHRAGM]
7) EXHALE GENTLY, FULLY, WITH PER-
FECT CONTROL, SQUEESING OUT THE
LAST POSSIBLE BIT OF AIR.
IT IS DURING EXHALATION THAT THE
MAGNETIC AND ELECTRIC AND THER-
MAL FORCES BLEND AND TRAVEL TO THE
OUTER RING „PASS NCT‚‚ AND THEN RETURN
CAUSING ECSTASY AND INTENSE CALM
AND POISE, THIS IS CALLED RECHAKA [HINDOO]
IN YOGAH, WHILE THE INHALATION IS
CALLED PURAKA.
  PHENOMENA AND CAUTION.
YOU WILL FEEL HEAT WAVES AND ELECTRIC
SHOCKS AT THE BASE OF THE SKULL, AND
IN THE CEREBELLUM AND INTER-BRAIN
AND MAGNETIC CURRENT FLOW ALONG

THE SPINE UPWARD INTO THE MEDULLA
OBLONGATA, CORPORA QUADRIGENIA,
FIFTH AND FOURTH VENTRICLES, CORPUS
CALLO██████, CORPORA STRATA, PONS
VAROLLI, PITUITIARY GLAND OR BODY
THIRD VENTRICLE AND PINEAL GLAND
OR HYPOPHYSIS (PITUITIARY IS EPIPHYSIS)
ALSO IN SEPTUM LUCIDUM AND OTHER
PARTS, YOU WILL HEAR A PULSATING SOUND
LIKE A BELL OR CHIME AND FEEL PUL-
SATIONS WITH A SENSE OF SWELLING
OR EXPANSION OF AURA, AND SOME-
TIMES A FEELING AS IF BEATING
OR FOLDING OF WINGS, OF MOVING
AS IF A BIRD WAS CLASPED TO THE
BACK OF THE SKULL OR HEAD, — THIS
IS THE KA OR BIRD (BA) OF THE
EGYPTIAN MYTHOLOGY.
THIS IS ALL RIGHT, BUT WHEN THINGS
SUDDENLY GO DARK, YOU STOP, OR
IF YOU CONTINUE, REMEMBER THAT
YOU WILL GO INTO A SLEEP OR TRANCE
STATE, AND MUST NOT BE DISTUR-
BED UNTIL YOUR GUARDIAN ANGEL
OR HEAVENLY FATHER AWAKENS
YOU, — ALSO IF YOUR KNEES RISE
FROM THE FLOOR OR BODY RISES IN THE
AIR, STOP AT ONCE. —
YOU DO NOT WANT LEVITATION TO OCCUR

— THE TRANCE STATE HOWEWER IS HEA-
-LING, AND GIVES THE POWER OF LAYING
ON OF HANDS OR HEALING BY SO DOING.

8) WHILE EXHALING RELAX GRIP ON
BARS OR STAFFS, BUT LET HANDS
GRASP GENTLY AND HOLD TO THEM (BARS
STAFFS).   I u

REMAIN ON KNEES OR SEATED FOR
THREE (3) MINUTES AND (12) TWELVE
SECONDS AFTER COMPLETE EXERCISE.

FULL EXERCISE IS (8) EIGHT BREATHS
OF TWENTY FOUR (24) SECONDS EACH
[INHALATION 7 SEC. HOLD 7 SEC. EXHALATION
7 SEC. HOLD 3 SEC.] - 192 SECOND OR (3)
THREE MINUTES (12) TWELVE SECONDS.

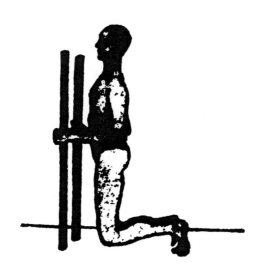

THE TRANSMUTATION TRANSFORMATION
AND TRANSFIGURATION EXERCISE, THIS
IS CALLED ROSICRUCIAN PHILOSOPHERS
STONE FOR THE TRANSMUTATION OF
BASE ELEMENTS INTO GOLD, ALSO
THE TRANSFIGURATION IN THE GARDEN
OF GATRA-SA-MARA - AND OF THE
TRANSFORMATION OF THE ELECTRIC
AND MAGNETIC FORCES AND POWERS
OF THE INDIVIDUAL AND UNIVERSAL SO
AS TO BLEND THE AURIC SPHERES OR
"EGGS" OF MAN AND EARTH INTO ONE,
- THIS BRINGS UNIFICATION OR
AT ONENES - ATONEMENT AND
IS THE EGYPTIAN "AT-UN" - IT
BRINGS ONE INTO COMMUNION WITH
THE DIVINE, ANGELIC, CELESTIAL,
HEAVENLY, HUMAN AND AURICAL,
BLENDED INTO HARMONIUS ACCORD
THRU MUSIC, SOUND, MAGNETIC
AND ELECTRIC FIELDS OF CONTACT;

NOTE: DURING THE EXERCISE DO NOT HAVE ANY
CHAIRS, TABLES OR OBJECS STANDING AROUND
BECAUSE IF GOING IN TRANCE YOU MAY
FALL AND STRIKE OBJECTS WITH YOUR HEAD
HURTING YOURSELF. IT IS ADVISABLE TO HAVE
PILLOWS AND RUGS THROWN ABOUT.

VII (SEVENTH) MASTER·ARCANE.
[EXERCISE]·(WEATHER CONTROL).

THIS EXERCISE IS A SEPARATE ONE CALLED
THE SEVENTH ARCANE, BUT HAVING IN
ITSELF A SEPARATE PLACE AS A PURELY
MAGICAL WORK, CONNECTED WITH WEATHER
CONTROL.—

∴. STAND ERECT (2) TWO FEET AWAY FROM
A STAND OR A ALTAR, ON WHICH THERE
IS A SQUARE, ROUND, PENTAGONAL OR
OTHER FORM OF WESSEL, ABOUT TWO(2
FEET IN DIAMETER, AND SIX(6) INCHES
HIGH, FILLED HALF WITH PURE WATER
— THE STAND SHOULD BE OF HEIGHT
PERMITTING PUTTING OF HANDS ON TOP
OF IT WITHOUT BENDING OR STRAINING.
FACE IN THE DIRECTION OF THE SUN,
OR MOON, OR STARS, ACCORDINGLY.
NOW CLEANSE THE LUNGS BY PANTING
TROWING OUT ALL RESIDUAL AIR.

SUBMERGE THE HANDS IN WESSEL WITH
WATER, PALMS RESTNG ON THE BOTTOM
OF IT, FINGERS SPREAD FANLIKE,
THUMBS AND FOREFINGERS OF BOTH
HANDS TOUCHING EACH OTHER UNDER
WATER.

INHALE DEEPLY FOR 7 (SEVEN) SECONDS
HOLD 1 (ONE SECOND), AND EXHALE
THRU THE MOUTH, SLOWLY, SOUNDING
A SIGH, UNTIL THE AIR IS OUT FROM
THE LUNGS. VOICE SHOULD SOUND LIKE

37

DEEP SIGH. [EXHALATIONS ARE TIMED ONLY
TO MAKE THEM RUN NATURALY AND EASILY
WITHOUT PRESCRIBED 7 SECONDS].
(1) ONE SECOND STOP, INHALE AGAIN FOR
(7) SEVEN SECONDS, STOP (1) ONE SECOND,
AND EXHALE THRU THE MOUTH WITH
A MOANING SOUND, LIKE MOANING,
AND AT THE SAME TIME WHISTLING.
THE STOP (1) ONE SECOND, AGAIN INHALE
DEEPLY FO (7) SEVEN SECONDS, STOP (1)
ONE SECOND, AND EXHALE THRU THE
MOUTH WITH A ROARING SOUND, LIKE
ROARING OF THE WIND, MIXED WITH
WHISTLING OF IT.
THOSE ARE THE THREE (3) COMPLETE
BREATS — SIGHING, MOANING AND
ROARING. -
REPEAT THEM FOUR TIMES, MAKING
TOTAL OF (12) TWELVE BREATHS.
NOTE: THE IS A WORD WHICH IS TO BE
USED WITH, SIGHING, MOANING, AND
ROARING BREATHS, AND THIS WORD
FORM THE BACKGROUND FOR THEM,
GIVING THEM VIBRATION TO AVAKEN,
THE ELEMENTAL SPIRITS OF THE
WIND, STORM, HURRICANE E.T.C. —
THIS WORD IS —
∴J-HAU-HAA∴ TO BE INTERWOVEN
WITH THE EXHALATION OF THE AIR,
IN ▬▬▬▬▬ SIGHING, MOANING,
AND ROARING. THIS ARCANE THRU
ATTRACTING POWERS OF WIND AND

STORM, CHANGES SORROUNDING CLIMATIC
CONDITIONS, WITH HELP OF THE MIGHTY
SPIRITS - EL BORACH (SPIRIT OF THE LIGHT-
NING-) AND WAAT (SPIRIT OF THE WIND)":

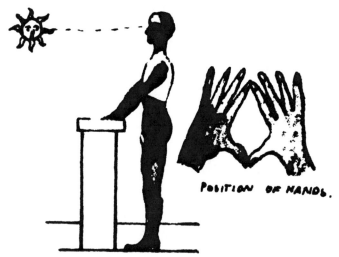

POSITION OF HANDS.

NOTE: EYES SHOLD BE FIXED, BUT VERY LIGHTLY,
SO THAT AT TIMES ONE IS ACTUALLY SEEING
ONLY BLURR.

∴ ALL THE PREVIUS COMPRISES THE SEVEN GREAT
ARCANES OF THE MASTER SYSTEM, THE SEVEN
KEYS OF ABSOLUTE LIBERATION FROM ADVERSE
SORROUNDINGS, INFLUENCES AND HEREDITARY
CHAINS, AND SLAVERY.-
THIS SHORT PATH, ESTABLISHES THE MASTER
RHYTM IN THE BODY, WHICH YOU MUST STRIVE
TO KEEP AS OFTEN AS YOU CAN (SEVEN SECONDS

39

INHALATION, ONE SECOND STOP, SEVEN SECONDS
EXHALATION, ONE SECOND STOP). THIS WILL PUT
YOU WITH THE GOOD THOUGHT, GOOD WORD AND
GOOD DEED, AND OPEN CHANNELS, ESTABLISHING
CONNECTIONS WITH THE MASTER THOUGHT,
AND HEAVENLY FATHER. YOU HAVE THEN
ALL THE KNOWLEDGE, ALL THE AUTHORITY,
AND ALL THE POWERS AND FORCES AT
YOUR COMMAND. YOU ARE ON THE PATH
AND YOUR GREAT TEACHER - THE HEAVENLY
FATHER WILL INSTRUCT YOU IN EVERYTHING
PERSONALLY, SO THAT YOU DO NOT NEED ANY
OTHER TEACHERS, OR HUMAN AUTHORI-
TIES.∴

GENERAL ∴ COMPENDIUM.

∴ IN THE WORK ON MASTERY THE MAIN
AND THE ONLY OBJECT IS TO ATTAIN COMMU-
NION WITH THE HARMONIOUS CREATIVE
POWER OF THE WORLD, AND CONSCIOUSLY
JOINING THE FORCES FOR SOLVING THE
DESTINIES OF THE EVOLUTION TOWARD
IMMORTAL ONENESS.
FIRST STEPS IN THIS PROCESS IS MASTERING
THOUGHT AND THRU IT MASTERING THE
BODY.
TO MASTER MEANS TO OVERPOWER, TO SUBDUE
TO RULE, TO KNOW; TO UNDERSTAND THO-
ROUGHLY, - IT MEANS ALSO DOMINION; SUPER
IORITY, VICTORY, OF BEINGS CONSCIOUS OF
IT. PROCESS OF DEVELOPEMENT IS CALLED
«THE GREAT WORK» AND IS CONSISTING OF
6/SIX GREAT MASTERARCANES CONSTITU-
TING THE «SHORT PATH» QUINTESSENCE

OF THE WAYS AND MEANS, FOR DEVELOPEMENT
OF CONSCIOUS MASTERY.
THE MAN IS GENERALLY IN A STATE OF
SLAVERY, PRODUCED BY IGNORANCE, ON
ONE OR MORE PLANES OF HIS ENTITY, I.E
PHYSICAL - MENTAL - SPIRITUAL AND
PSYCHIC; WHICH STATE COMES FROM THE
DIFFERENT MISLEAD IMPRESSIONS ON
THE HUMAN SYSTEM, LIKE PRECONCEIVING
AND CONCEVING STATE OF THE MOTHER-
PRENATAL INFLUENCE OF MOTHERS
THOUGHT, FEELING AND WILLING.
INFLUENCE OF THE MOMENT AND
MANNER OF BIRTH, WHICH HAS LOT
TO DO WITH LIFE CURRENTS CIRCULATING
IN THE BODY, AND WHICH IS OF GREAT
IMPORT IN HUMAN PERSONAL HISTORY.
   BIRTH OF A CHILD CAN BE COMPARED
TO TAKING A FISH OUT OF WATER INTO
THE AIR. - THE SORROUNDINGS ARE
CHANGED IN VERY GREAT EXTENT, AND
FIRST IMPRESSIONS MOULD THE DESTI-
NY, BY SHAPING AND PIERSING NEW
CHANNELS FOR ENERGIES AND LIFE
CURRENT. NOTE! AFTER BIRTH OF THE CHILD THE UMBILICUS
SHOULD BE CUT ONLY AFTER IT COLLAPSES 3 TIMES.
   NEXT COMES THE AGE OF CHILDHOOD,
PUBERTY, AND ADOLESCENCE OF SEVEN
YEARS EACH — DURING WHICH INFLUEN-
CES OFTEN ADVERSE IMPRINT THEMSELVES
UPON THE DEVELOPING ENTITY, WARP
ITS GROWTH, AND CREATING AT TIMES
UNNATURAL WAYS OF IMPRESSIONS AND
EXPRESSIONS.

41

THE PROCESS OF LIBERATION FROM THE BON-
DAGE OF SLAVERY OF DARKNESS AND IGNO-
RANCE COULD BE ONLY FORMULATED AND
BE GIVEN OUT BY THE SOULS WHO ATTAINED
THE FREDOM, AND WERE FILLED WITH PURE
LIGHT OF WISDOM AND UNDERSTANDING.—
IT WAS DONE BY THE MASTERS, AND
IS CALLED THE MASTER SYSTEM, FROM
ETERNITY INTO ETERNITY FOR THE GUI-
DING OF HUMAN RACE.

THE AEONS OF INVOLUTION, REVOLU-
TION AND EVOLUTION, THOUGHTS,—
—FEELING AND WILLING, THRU MANY
REBIRTHS—THRU PAIN—SUFFERING AND
WORK—A RACE PUREST WAS EVOLVED,
THE ██████████ RACE OF MASTERS AND
SAVIOURS.—

MAN IS THE CENTER IN WHICH
CURRENTS—POWERS AND FORCES OF THE
WORLD ARE CROSSING AND MERGING
TO FIND THRU HIM THE PERFECT EX-
PRESSION.

THE MASTER SYSTEM PROVES THAT
EVERYTHING IS ONE, BUILT FROM
THE SAME CLAY OF PRIMORDIAL ENER-
GY, IN DIFFERENT STATE OF VIBRATION
(SPEED OF POSITIVE AND NEGATIVE COMPONENTS
OF MATTER, WHICH (THE MATTER) IS CONDEN-
CED ENERGY—POSITIVE AND NEGATIVE IN
DIFFERENT PROPORTIONS AND STATES OF
DENSENESS.)—(POSITIVE IS MINUS WITHIN
THE VACUUM, NEGATIVE IS NEUTRALISING
PLUS IN THE VACUUM, TAKEN BY DIVISION
SPARK FROM NEUTRAL—WHICH IS VACUUM

42

THIS ONE WHICH IS ALSO TWO, WHICH
IS ALSO TWO WITH AGAIN ONE SORR-
OUNDING, WHICH IS THREE. - IS THE
  "THAT IS" AND IS CALLED THE —
∴GA-YA-LHA-MA∵.
THE HUMAN BODY ABSORBS THE GA-YA-
-LHA-MA THRU THE BREATH. AIR ENTERS
THE NOSE, BEING GIVEN SPIRAL MOTION BY
TURBINATES, AND ELONGATING INTO TWO
CONES STRIKING EACH OTHER AS THEY
MEET.

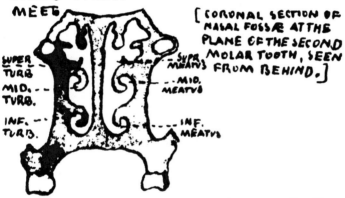

[CORONAL SECTION OF
NASAL FOSSÆ AT THE
PLANE OF THE SECOND
MOLAR TOOTH, SEEN
FROM BEHIND.]

UPER
TURB
MID.
TURB.
INF.
TURB.

SUPR
MEATUS
MID.
MEATUS
INF.
MEATUS

THE AIR IN PASSING GETS HEATED, AND
GOING THRU PHARYNX, RELEASES THE GA-
YA-LHA-MA WHICH SINKS THRU THE PHA
RYNX BEHIND THE SOFT PALATE IN THE
PROXIMITY OF TWELVE NERVE AND FIRST PAIR
OF CERVICAL NERVES, IN THE PROXIMITY OF ME-
DULLA OBLONGATA, NINTH, TENTH, AND ELEVENTH
NERVES. AIR THEN GOES TO THE LUNGS WHERE
IT OXYDISES THE BLOOD.
GA-YA-LHA-MA HAS FOUR STATES OF VIBRA-
TION, HAVING DISTINCT COLOUR VIBRATIONS
AND AREAS WHERE IT IS STORED IN THE BODY.

43

FILLING WITH ENERGIES IS DONE SIMULTA-
NEUSLY IN TWO PLACES IN THE BODY, BOTH
OF THEM BEING CHARED AT THE SAME TIME
DURING THE PERIOD OF EXHALATION.
THE FOUR STATES OF VIBRATION OF 'GA-YA-
-LHA-MA, AND CORRESPONDING COLOURS,
WITH THE PARTS TO BE CHAGED IN THE
BODY ARE:—

1) PHYSICAL — COLOUR RED (VERMILLION), PARTS
OF THE BODY TO BE CHARGED — LOWER PART
OF THE STOMACH AND BACK OF THE HEAD.

2) MENTAL (INTELLECTUAL) - COLOUR - YELLOW
(CHROME), PARTS OF THE BODY TO BE CHAR-
GED — CHEST AND FOREHEAD.

3) SPIRITUAL (DYNAMIC) - COLOUR - BLUE (ULTRA-
MARINE), PARTS OF THE BODY TO BE CHAR-
GED — UPPER PART OF THE ABDOMEN (SOLAR
PLEXUS) AND TOP OF THE HEAD.

4) PSYCHIC - COLOUR WHITE ! WHICH IS MIXTURE
OF RED-YELLOW-BLUE), PARTS OF THE BODY
TO BE CHARGED - LEGS, FORELEGS, FEET
AND ARMS, FOREARMS, HANDS, AND FACE.
(IN CERTAIN CASES THE COLOUR FOR PSYCHIC
IS BLACK.).

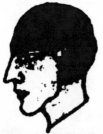

CURRENTS OF GA-YA-
-LHAMA CHARGING
THE HEAD.

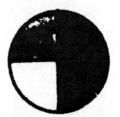

THE ANCIENT REPRE-
SENTATION OF THE GA-
-YA-LHA-MA CURRENTS
ACCORDING TO THE STAGES
OF VIBRATION IN THE
HUMAN HEAD.

CURRENTS OF GA-YA-LHA-MA CHARGING THE
BODY.-

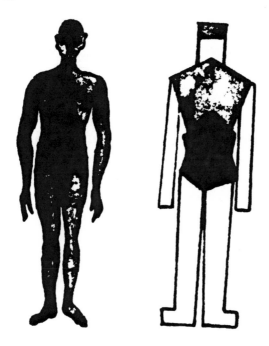

:o STAR WHCHIS
THE CROWN, THE
POWER, THE LOVE
THE FIVE POINTS
OF FELLOWSHIP,
STAR OF RESSU-
RECTION.

∴THE STAR OF MAN.
THE STAR OF SAVIOUR.
THE STAR OF SENSES.
THE MORNING STAR.
THE BRIGHTEST STAR.
THE STAR OF WISEMEN.
THE STA OF ELEMENTS∴

PENTAGRAM OF THE MAN (MICROCOS-
MOS MIRRORING THE MACROCOSMOS),
THE SECRET OF THE SACRED MASTERY
AND SUPREMACY.

NATURE'S INNERMOST SECRETS ARE WAITING
TO BE COMMANDED BY MASTERS, TO WORK
FOR THE BENEFIT OF THE WORLD.

BOOKS OF ZEND AVESTA, DECLARE
THE MASTERY AND ANSWER THE RIDLE
OF HUMAN LIFE:- WHY I AM HERE ?
".'. I AM ON THIS EARTH—TO RECLAIM
THE EARTH,—TO TURN THE DESERTS
INTO PARADISE,—A PARADISE
MOST SUITABLE TO GOD AND HIS
ASSOCIATES TO DWELL THEREIN.'.

THIS IS TRUE GOAL OF LIFE. SOUL THAT
REALISES THIS TRUTH CONSCIOUSLY,
STANDS ON THE PATH AS THE MASTER
AND SAVIOUR.

GOOD THOUGHT, GOOD WORD AND GOOD DEED,
ARE ANALOGOUS WITH MASTER THOUGHT,
MASTER WORD AND MASTER DEED, EXPRE-
SSIONS WITH THE ASPECTS OF AHU-RA-
-MAZ-DA. [LIGHT]

BAD THOUGHT, BAD WORD AND BAD DEED,
ARE ANALOGOUS WITH SLAVE THOUGHT,
SLAVE WORD AND SLAVE DEED, EXPRE-
SSIONS WITH THE ASPECTS OF ANGRO-
-MAINOUS. (ANGRY-MIND)[DARKNESS]

THE MASTER SYSTEM TEACHES
THAT THRU THE CONSCIOUS CONTROL
OF THE BREATH, AND ESTABLISHING
THE MASTER RHYTM THRU SYSTEM
OF EXERCISES, CALLED ARCANES, WE
CHANGE OUR IMPRESSIONS AND EXPRE-
SSIONS—FROM SLAVERY INTO MASTERY.

47

BE CONSCIOUS AND POSITIVE, ASSERT YOUR
TRUE I - YOUR TRUE EGO, RENOUNCE THE
BONDAGE OF TIES AND SLAVERY, AND DECLA-
RE - THE MASTERY.
THE SIGN OF MASTER SYSTEM IS, WHEN
YOU MEET ANOTHER HUMAN BEING, STAND
STRAIGHT, (ERECT) SPINE STRAIGHT, SHOULDERS
BACK, CHEST FORWARD, HEAD UP, CHIN IN,
GASE QUIET, LEVEL WITH THE EYES.
RIGHT FOOT FORWARD, FORMING A SLIGHT
ANGLE WITH THE LEFT. (V). (MASTER BREATH)
WHEN YOU SIT, SIT ERECT, GASE LEVEL
WITH THE EYES.) HEAD UP CHIN IN. LEGS RE-
LAXED FEET, FORELEGS AND TIGHS FORMING
LETTER V. (MASTER BREATH.)

∴ YAT-HA-AH-HU-VAI-RIO∴ - THE WILL
OF THE LORD IS THE LAW OF RIGHTEUS-
NESS.

"YAT-HA-AH-HU-VO-" THE WILL OF THE
LORD IS POWER (LIGHTNING THAT STRIKES)
WE ARE MYSTERIOUS MIRROR, WHICH
IN ITS PURE STATE REFLECTS THE WOR-
LD, ITS CASES AND EFFECTS,
IF THEN INSIDE OF YOU, YOU CREAT THE
CAUSE, EFFECT WILL FOLLOW = AND BE
REFLECTED THRU THE MIRROR OF THE SOUL
-INTO ANY MEDIUM BECOMING FLESH.
(REFLECTION IS POLARISED, WHILE THE
RAYS BEFORE STRIKING THE REFLECTING
SURFACE ARE MORE IN THE STATE OF
CHAOS.) - ALWAYS STRIKE AT THE CAUSES,

48

CHANGING THEM, AND THE EFFECTS WILL
FOLLOW.
∴ STATE OF MASTERSHIP IS TO BE
AT ALL TIMES CONSCIOUSLY, AND IN
POSITIVE RECEPTIVE ATTITUDE, OPEN
TO ALL GOOD AND POSITIVE POWERS TO
FLOW THRU YOU. — AND TO DIRECT
THEM IN THE PROPER CHANNELS OF
GOOD THOUGHT, GOOD WORD AND GOOD
DEED ∴
THOSE TITANIC POWERS ARE EVERY-
WHERE, SORROUNDING US AT ALL TIMES
— BEING THE EMANATIONS OF GOD,
AND ALWAYS SEEKING THE ENTRANCE
INTO OUR BEINGS, TO EXPRESS THEM-
SELVES THRU US.
TO BE RECEPTIVE TO THOSE POWERS —
— IS TO ESTAGLIH MASTER RHYTM IN
US AND RELINQUISH THE MOTHERS
IMPRESSION IN THE TIME OF CONCEPTION,
AND PREGNANCY, AND DEFEAT THE
BRAND OF ADVERSE SORROUNDINGS,
COINCIDENCES AND INFLUENCES.
IN THE ANCIENT MYSTERIES, ESTA-
BLISHING OF THE MASTER BREATH
AND MASTER RHYTM, WAS DONE BY
THE FOUR GREAT INITIATIONS OF THE
ELEMENTS.
1) FIRST INITIATION WAS BY WATER.
SUBMERSION IN COLD WATER, AFFEC-
TING THYROID, BROUGHT ABOUT A
SPASM, WHICH WHEN CORRECTLY
DONE ESTABLISHED THE MASTER
VIBRATION IN THE BODY.

THIS WAS INITIATION OF MOSES AND CHRIST,
AND USED IN THIS DAY IN CHRISTIAN CHURCH.
2) THE SECOND INITIATION WAS BY FIRE.
THE NEOPHITE PASSING BETWEEN TWO FIRES
OR GOING THRU FIRE, HAD TO HOLD HIS
BREATH, FOR THE IMPOSSIBILITY TO INHALE
THE SMOKE. (BABYLONIAN AND DRAVIDIAN
MYSTERIES).
3) THE THIRD INITIATION WAS BY AIR, DROPING
DOWN FROM A HEIGHT IN SPECIALLY PRE-
PARED CONTRIVANCES. THIS PROCESS
AFFECTED THE BREATH AND SOLAR
PLEXUS. (EGYPTIAN MYSTERIES, ALSO
CHRIST PUT BY SATAN ON THE MOUNTAIN
AND THEN THROWN FROM IT).
4) THE FOURTH INITIATION WAS BY EARTH,
GETTING BODY COVERED WITH EARTH, BEING
BURRIED ALIVE FOR CERTAIN PERIOD OF TIME,
ALSO LISTENING TO THE (SILENCE) IN SUBTE-
RENIAN CAVES, TO GET THE SACRED RHYTM
OF THE EARTS HEART, WHICH VIBRATES
IN UNISON AND HARMONY WITH THE UNIVERCE.
(HEART OF THE EARTH COTRACTS FOR SEVEN
SECOND, ONE SECOND PAUSE, SEVEN SECONDS
EXPANDS, ONE SECOND STOP) THIS IS THE
SACRED MASTER RHYTM.)
   THOSE ARE THE GREATH FOUR INITIA-
TIONS IN THE MYSTERIES OF MASTERY.
   IN THE MASTER SYSTEM THERE ALWAYS
WAS THE SIMPLIFIED, CONDENSED AND
CORRECT-MANNER OF DISCLOSING THE
TEACHINGS AND ARCANES OF MASTERY,
BUT IT IS ALWAYS GIVEN ONLY FOR THE
SUFFICIENTLY DEVELOPED AND REA-
DY CANDITATES, AND IN CASES OF

EVOLVED, WORTHY AND WELL QUALIFIED
SOULS.
THOSE ONLY HEAR THE CALL WHO ARE
READY, TO THE OTHERS MOMENT DID NOT
ARIVED YET, BUT SOMETIME THROUGH
OUT ETERNITY IT WILL.
THE MASTER SYSTEM IS SOLVING
EVERY PROBLEM, IN EVERY DE-
PARTAMENT OF LIFE, IS ANSVERING
EVERY QUESTION, AND MEETS
EVERY SITUATION — ON THE PHYSICAL,
—MENTAL, SPIRITUAL AND PSYCHIC
PLANES.
IT IS DOING ALL THE THINGS THAT
THE OTHER SYSTEMS CLAIM TO DO, THAT
HAVE BEEN BORROWING FROM IT
    MASTER SYSTEM MEANS THAT WHEN
IT IS THOUGHT FULLY AND COMPLETELY
EVERYWHERE, ALL THE OTHER SYSTEMS
WILLBE SHOWN TO BE WHAT THEY ARE,
THAT IS THAT THEY WERE ALWAYS FAL-
LING BELOW THE STANDART OF FIRST
AND THE ONLY WORD OF MASTERS
OF ARIAS, FROM ETERNITY INTO
ETERNITY.
    WE WILL DEFINE HERE WHAT IS MYSTICISM,
OCCULTISM AND MAGICK,
① MYSTICISM IS CAREFUL OBSERVATION THRU
  SUPERSENSITIVE CHANNELS OF IMPRE-
  SSIONS. (
② OCCULTISM IS CORRECT INTERPRETATION,
  THRU APPLYING OF THE CONSCIOUS DISCRIMI-
  NATION OF THE SOUL.
③ MAGICK IS PRACTICAL APPLICATION OF
  SUPERSENSITIVE OBSERVATION AND INTER-

51

PRETATION. IT IS TO MAKE THINGS APPEAR
DISAPPEAR AND CHANGE ONE THING INTO
THE OTHER. - CREATION, DESTRUCTION AND
TRANSMUTATION.

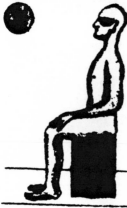

∴ SITTING MASTER
SYSTEM POSTURE∵

∴ POSTURE CALLED-POSI-
TIVE IN RELAXED ATTI-
TUDE, TO RECEIVE, ANA-
LISE AND DIRECT CON-
SCIOUSLY, IMPRESSIONS
AND EXPRESSIONS, ACCOR-
DING TO THE LAW, AND
SPIRIT OF THE TIMES∵

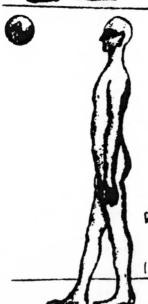

∴ STANDING MASTER
SYSTEM POSTURE∵

∴ UPRIGHT AND ON THE
LEVEL∵

STANDING LIKE A MEN
IN MASTER SYSTEM.
POSITIVE IN RELAXED
ATTITUDE.
RIGHT FOOT FORWARD
DENOTES SUN CURRENT
RA) POSITIVE AND ELECTRIC.

[LEFT FOOT FORWARD
WOULD MEAN MOUN-
(MA) NEGATIVE AND MAG-
NETIC

52

LESSER ARCANES AND GREAT

EXERCISES FOR DIFFERENT PARTICULAR
PURPOSES, ACCORDING TO MASTER SYSTEM

I.L. ARCANE. <u>DOCTRINE OF THE HEART</u>

OLDEST SYMBOL - SWASTIKA REPRE-
SENTS CONTRACTING OF THE HEART,
WHILE SOUWASTICA - EXPANING.
DIVIDING THE WORK IN MYSTICISM AND
OCCULTISM AND MAGICK INTO TWO DISTINCT
PATHS. - I (FIRST- DOCTRINE OF THE CLOSED
HEART - BUT OPEN MIND - DEVELOPING
REASON - IT IS SYMBOL OF SOUWASTICA. USED
IN THE ORIENT,). II (SECOND - DOCTRINE OF
THE OPEN HEART - AND FEELINGS, BRINGS
IN WISDOM - IT IS SYMBOL OF SWASTIKA.
USED IN OXIDENT.)

(CROSS SECTION OF THE HEART WILL SHOW
THE MUSCLES IN THE FORM OF SWASTIKA
AND SOUWASTIKA, CONTRACTING AND
EXPANDING THE HEART.)
THE DOCTRINE OF THE HEART, IS ONE OF
THE GREATEST SIGNS OF THE FULFILMENT
AND EVOLUTION IT IS THE DEVELOPEMENT
OF LOVE AND DISCRIMINATION, AND IT
PENETRATES ALL THE SECRET AND SACRED
TRADITIONS. OF THE WHITE RACE.

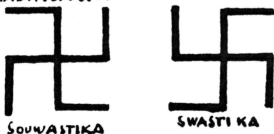

SOUWASTIKA   SWASTIKA

53

SIT DOWN IN A QUIET PLACE FACING SUN,
MOON OR PLANET (IN THE DIRECTION), BREATH
DEEPLY, THEN RELAX, AND WITHDRAW
WITHIN YOURSELF.

FOLD YOUR HAND LAVING ONLY TWO FINGERS
OUTSTRETCHED, INDEX AND MIDDLE (DESTINY
AND TEACHER), AND APPLY THEM TOWARD
THE HEART. WATCH THE HEART BEAT, AND
CONSCIOUSLY FILL IT WITH LOVE, REPEA-
TING THE WORD "LOVE" WITH EVERY
HEART BEAT. (WORD "LOB" CAN BE USED
FROM WHICH DERIVES WORD "LOVE"—
ONE OF THE TWO SOUNDS OF THE HEART;
—SYSTOLE AND DIASTOLE — LOB AND DOB.
GRADUALLY YOU BECAME CONSCIOUS OF
THE FEELING OF LOVE CONCENTATING IN
THE HEARTH, SENSATION OF CONGESTION
WHICH IS PRESSURE OF FEELING AND
FULLNESS IN THE CARDIAC REGION.

WHEN FEELING REACHES ITS PINNACLE
OF TENSION, COVER THE RIGHT HAND
GENTLY WITH THE LEFT, AND SLOWLY
WITHDRAW THE RIGHT HAND FROM UNDER
THE LEFT AT THE SAME TIME SHAPING
LEFT HAND WITH FOREFINGER AND
MIDDLE FINGER POINTING TO THE
HEART, THE OTHER FINGER CLOSED.

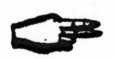 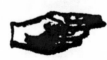

∴ WAY OF
CLOSING HANS.
(CALLED ALSO
SACERDOTAL
HAND!

WITH EVERY HEART BEAT UTTER WORD
AL—IM, THIS IS THE HOLY WORD WHICH
OPENS THE HEART. THE WORD IS REPEA,
TED WITH BEATS OF THE HEART, AND
YOU ENTER THE INTERIOR OF THE HEART,
FILLED WITH RED CLOUDS AND MIST,
IN THE CENTER IS STANDING THE ARC,
WITH MEASURES OF DISCRIMINATION,
AND OVER THE ARC YOU SEE THE BLAZING
PENTAGRAM, WITH THE ALL SEING
EYE IN THE CENTER.
YOU WORSHIP THEN AND COMMUNE,
AND SEND OUT LOVE, TO UNDERSTAND,
REACH, HELP AND BLESS.
THEN HAVING ENDED, YOU PUT THE
RIGHT HAND LIKE IN THE BEGINNING
OF THE ARCANE AND WITHDRAW THE
LEFT HAND, AND WITH INDEX FINGER
AND MIDDLE ON THE HEART REPEAT
WITH EVERY BEAT OF THE HEART
WORD „PEACE", TO FILL THE HEART
WITH IT.

LOVE

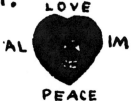
AL   IM

PEACE

THIS COMPLETES THE DOCTRINE OF THE
SACRED HEART.
NOTE. HEART SHOLD BE CONSULTED IN EVERY
IMPORTANT UNDERTAKING, BY PUTTING ON
IT THE TWO FINGERS OF THE LEFT HAND,
IT ALSO IS USED IN HEALING.

55

II G. ARCANE. <u>CREATION EXERCISE.</u>

USED FOR - AWAKENING OF THE DESIRE,
AND TRANSMUTING IT INTO WILL POWER
STAND ERECT, SPINE STRAIGHT HEAD
UP CHIN IN. RELAX AND BREATH
DEEPLY.

PUT YOUR HANDS OVER SOLAR PLEXUS,
ON THE PART WHERE IS ENSIFORM CAR-
TILAGE. HOLD THEM THERE LIGHTLY,
THINK OF THE THING THAT YOU DESIRE,
AND SLIGHTLY HOLDING THE BREATH,
SHAKE DIAPHRAGM WITH SHORT SPAS-
MODIC MOVEMENTS, SOMETIMES LET-
TING THE BREATH IN, OR OUT, WHILE
VIBRATING, UNTIL YOU WILL FEEL
THE HUNGER AND PANG OF THE DESIRE
IN YOUR SOLAR PLEXUS, OFTEN ALSO
FELT LIKE HEAT.

THAN RELAX ABSOLUTELY THE ABDOMINAL
MUSCLES AND EXHALE ALL THE AIR FROM
THE LUNGS PRESSING THE FINGERS OF
BOTH HANDS DEEP INTO THE STOMACK
AT THE STERNUM PART (ENSIFORM
CARTILAGE) BETWEEN THE RIBS.
WHEN DOING THIS LOWER YOUR HEAD
UNTIL THE CHIN WILL REST ON THE CHEST.
(ALL THE EXERCISE DONE WITH EYES HALF
CLOSE, INTROSPECTIVE GAZE)
AFTER EXHALING ALL THE AIR, HOLD
FOR SEVEN SECONDS PRESSING HANDS
STRONGLY INTO THE STOMACK, WITH
VIBRATING PRESSURE, AND ALSO PRE-
SSING THE CHIN INTO THE CHEST, CONCEN

TRATING OF FEELING OF TAKING HOLD
OF THE DESIRE, AS OF A REAL LIVING
THING.
NEXT BEGIN TO INHALE SLOWLY,
GRADUALLY LIFTING THE HEAD, BUT
NOT RELAXING THE DIGGING PRESSURE
ON THE SOLAR PLEXUS.
INHALE TO THE CAPACITY OF THE LUNGS
LIFTING THE HEAD, UNTIL IT WILL BE
LIFTED, LIKE FOR LOOKING UPWARD,
FOR PRAING.
THEN LOCK THE THROAT, SO THAT
THE AIR WONT ESCAPE. GIVE THE
AIR COMPRESSED IN THE LUNGS A
DOWNWARD SHOWE AGAINST THE
DIAPHRAGM, SOLAR PLEXUS AND
FINGERS OF HAND PRESSING AGAINST
IT. PRESSURE SHOULD THROW OF DIGGING
FINGERS WITH A SNAP.
THEN STOP PRESSING HANDS AGAINST
THE STOMACH, YOU ARE IN THE SUBCON-
SCIOUS AND SUPER CONSCIOUS STATE AND
CAN USE YOUR HANDS AND BODY WHEN
NECESSARY. YOU ARE IN THIS STATE
ALL THE TIME YOU HOLD YOUR BREATH
LOCKING THE THROAT IS REPRESEN-
TED AS CRUX ANSATA IN EGYPT,
NOOSE IN INDIA TIBET, TIE THAT BINDS
IN PERSIA E.TC.
PROCESS OF LOCKING THE THROAT AND
SHIFTING PRESSURE AGAINST THE
DIAPHRAGM, GIVES IN THE SOLAR
PLEXUS SUDDEN JOLT, SENDING SPI-
RITUAL ENERGY OF LONGING AND

DESIRE THRU THE SPINAL COLUMN UP-
WARDS TO THE BRAIN, IT IS FELT LIKE
HEAT AND PRESSURE MOUNTING WITHIN
THE SPINE, STRIKING PINEAL GLAND
(MEDULLA OBLONGATA), WHERE IT IS
FELT LIKE A SNAP, THEN REACHING
FORWARD, BEETWEN THE EYE BROWS,
WITH ANOTHER SNAP, AND FINALLY
THE TOP OF THE HEAD.
FEELING OF TENSION PERWADES THE
HEAD, THOUGHTS DISSAPEAR ONE
AFTER THE OTHER, SQUISED OUT OF THE
BRAIN, ONLY THOUGHT OF THE DESIRE
BLENDS WITH IT AND PERWADES THE
BRAIN THRU THE EGO GETTNG TRANS-
MUTED INTO THE WILL POWER, WHICH
CONNECTS DESIRE TO THE OBJECT OF THE
DESIRE, TAKING POSSESSION OF IT AND
MAKING IT COME THRU.

NOTE: FACE SUN,
MOON, PLANETS OF
STARS ACCORDING
TO THINGS YOU WORK
FOR ".

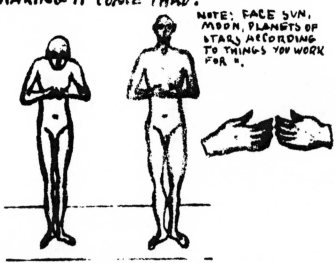

58

SYMBOLLICALLY REPRESENTED PROCESS
OF CREATION IS IN CADUCEUS OF HERMES
WITH THE TWO SERPENTS ENCIRCLING IT
MOUNTING TOWARD PINE CONE OR MER-
CURY'S HEAT WITH WINGS SPREAD ATTA-
CHED TO IT. ALSO WINGED SCARAB OF
THE EGYPTIANS, SKARAB REPRESENTING
HUMAN SKULL. IN ORIENT A SKULL, THE
SAME SYMBOL OFTEN USED IN CHRISTIAN
SYMBOLIC ART.
MERCURY (HERMES) CARRYING DEMAND
OR ORDER ON THE WINGS OF WILL.
   NOTE. THIS IS A GREAT ARCANE
(HERMETIC), AND USES SAME POWERS
CONSCIOUSLY DIRECTED, AS ARE AWENED
IN (6) (SIXTH MASTER ARCANE (EXERCISE)
IT IS USED IN EVERYTHING OF IMPOR
TANCE, IT MATERIALISES THINGS YOU
WANT, CURES DISEASES YOURS AND OTHERS
WILL MAKE YOU INSENSIBLE TO PAIN
(SELF ANASTHESIA) AND WILL PUT YOU
IN TRANCE, CATALEPTIC STATE OR
IN LETARGIC (HIBERNATING) CONDITION
IT AROUSES THE SERPENT POWER OF THE
BODY (KUNDALINI IN YOGA).
CAUTION: WORKING THOSE POWERS IS
BEST BEGINNING DELICATELY, AND BEING
IN PRACTICE WITH MAJOR MASTER ARCA-
NES.
WHEN GOING IN SUBCONSCIOUS OR SUPER-
CONSCIOUS STATE, WHILE IN IT YOUR EYES
GET OUT OF FOCUS, AND YOU SEE OBJECTS
DIMLY. THIS IS NORMAL AND TO BE
EXPECTED IN THIS POWERFUL EXERCISE
OF MASTERS, RULERS AND HIGH PRIESTS.
   CONVERGE

III G. ARCANE. PROJECTING OF POWER.
∴ RITUAL OF PENTAGRAM ∴ MASTER PROJECTION

THIS IS A PROJECTION OF POWER, DONE TO
BUILD THE WALL OF ABSOLUTE PROTECTION
AGAINST ADVERSE POWERS AND THOUGHTS
AND ALSO A POWERFUL AND TERRIBLE
WEAPON TO STRIKE AND DESTROY THE
ENEMIES.

FACE NORTH, - BEGIN BY DOING THE
TWELVE COMPLE BREATHS LIKE IN
THE FIRST (I) MASTER ARCANE, SITTING
AND USING MASTER BREATH SEVEN (7)
SECOND INHALATION, ONE (1) SECOND
STOP, SEVEN SECONDS EXHALATION,
(1) ONE SECOND STOP — TWELVE TIMES.

SET UP AND STAND UPRIGHT HEAD UP,
CHIN IN, RIGHT FOOT FORWARD, LIKE IN THE
SECOND (II) MASTER ARCANE. INHALE DEEP
NOW MOVE YOUR RIGHT ARM TO THE LEFT,
HAND CLOSED WITH INDEX FINGER POINTING,
FROM YOUR LEFT SIDE MAKE SWINGINLY A
STROKE UPWARD TO THE APEX OF THE PEN-
TAGRAM THAT YOU ARE BULDING, WHICH
WILL BE STRAIGHT OVER YOUR HEAD.
THAN SWING THE ARM DOWNWARD TO-
WARD THE RIGHT SIDE, BUILDING THIS
WAY FIRST UPPER CORNER OF THE PENTA-
GRAM, THEN SWING THE ARM TOWARD
DE LEFT SHOULDER, THEN HORISONTALLY
OVER THE RIGHT SHOULDER THAN BRING
THE ARM DOWN FROM UPPER RIGHT
SIDE TOWARD LOVER LEFT WHICH MO-
TION IS CLOSING THE PENTAGRAM,

WITHOUT STOPPING SWING THE ARM IN A
WIDE CIRCLE, AFTER ESCRIBING WHICH
CONTINUE MAKING HALF A CIRCLE TO-
WARD THE CENTER AT THE SAME
TIME STEPPING FORWARD WITH THE
RIGHT FOOT, AND MAKING A RHRUST
WITH THE ARM AND HAND, FOREFINGER
POINTING. (ACTUALLY THE CIRCLE AND
HALF A CIRCLE FORM A SPIRAL DRAWN
IN THE AIR FROM LEFT TO RIGHT.)
NOTE (ALL THE EXERCISE IS DONE POINTING
THE INDEX FINGER AS IF WRITING IN THE
AIR.)

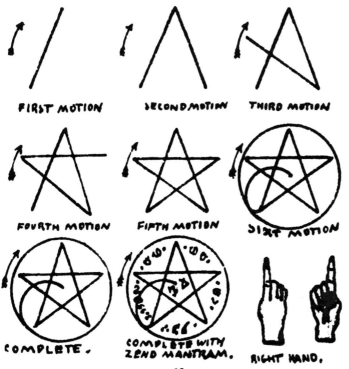

FIRST MOTION   SECOND MOTION   THIRD MOTION

FOURTH MOTION   FIFTH MOTION   SIXT MOTION

COMPLETE.   COMPLETE WITH ZEND MANTRAM.   RIGHT HAND.

WHEN BUILDING THE PENTAGRAM IN THE
AIR, SING THE SACRED WORD „YAT-HA-
AH-HU-VO"! WITH FIRST MOTION SING
„YAT", WITH THE SECOND-„HA", WITH
THE THIRD-„AH", WITH THE FOURTH-
-„HU", WITH THE FIFTH-„VO", WHEN
DOING SPIRAL AND THRUST SOUND
„OM" WITH ALL THE REST OF THE BREATH
USED ON THE END OF THE „OM" HUM-
MING SOUND.-
THEN DROP THE HAND AND ARM RELA-
XED TO THE SIDE.
PROJECT IT ACCORDING TO NESSESITY,
UP TO TWELWE TIMES, AND ALWAYS
FACING NORTH.
TO BUILD PROTECTIVE WALL YOU CAN MAKE
IT TO THE FOUR CORNERS OF THE EARTH,
ABOVE AND BELOW, USING ONLY THE -
PENTAGRAM WITHOUT THE SPIRAL THRUST
„YAT-HA-AH-HU-VO" - THIS WORD MEA-
NS - „THE WILL OF THE LORD IS POWER"
IT IS THE WORD THAT ROOSTER KNOWS.
THE WORD „OM" IS THE WORD THA LION
ROARS.
CAUTION! USE THIS ONLY WHEN YOU
KNOW THAT IT IS THE ONLY WAY,
TO ACT IN ACCORDANCE WITH THE
SPIRIT OF THE LAW. ∴

∴ ʒﾉ ·ɔ◌·◌ʊ◌·◌◌·↻ɯ◌◌ ∴
∴ ◌ ʒ ∴

IV. L. ARCANE. EXITING THE LIFE ENERGY
: TO BE USED WHEN YOU ARE TIRED PHYSI-
CALLY, MENTALLY, SPIRITUALLY OR PSYCHI-
CALLY, - ALSO BEFORE ANY TASK, OR TO
BRING POWER TO FACE AUDIENCE OF
ONE OR MORE. IT BRINGS ALERTNESS
AND MAGNETIC AND ELECTRIC POWERS
OF THE BODY INTO PLAY, STRENGHTENS
THE PENETRATING QUALITY OF THE EYES,
IT IS A QUICK HELPING EXERCISE.
SITTING OR STANDING, RELAX COMPLE-
TELY, INHALE AND EXHALE DEEPLY
FEW TIMES, EXHALE THOROUGHLY,
SPINE ERECT, HEAD UP, NOW BEGIN
TO INHALE FOR (7) SEVEN SECONDS,
TENSING UPPER PART OF THE BODY, -
CHEST, SHOULDERS, ARMS, NECK, JAW,
FOREARMS AND HANDS. (FOLD THE
FINGERS.), THEN VIBRATE TENSED
MUSCLES HOLDING THE BREATH FOR
SEVEN (7) SECONDS. EXHALE QUICLY
RELAXING COMPLETELY, OPENING
MOUTH AND SAYING. "- HA -".
DO IT ONCE. -
THIS EXERCISE IS SENDING CURRENTS
TO PINEAL GLAND (MEDULLA OBLONGATA)
STIMULATING IT. - THIS IS THE SER-
PENT WITHIN THE SPINAL COLUMN, RAI-
SING HIS HEAD IN ATTENTION, AND
SWELLING IT.
NOTE!. YOU WILL HEAR IN THE EARS
SOUND LIKE OF SILVER CHAINS, WHEN
YOU TENSE YOUR JAW, WHICH IS TO BE
EXPECTED.

L. ARCANE. HEALING POWER.

TO HEAL THE WOUNDS, STOP BLEEDING,
REMOVE PAIN, AND SET IN HEALING PROCESS
IN THE ORGANS IN THE BODY. - GET EASY
ACCESS TO THE PART AFECTED YOURS OR
ANOTHER, BREATH DEEPLY FOR FEW MOME-
NTS, THEN HOLD YOUR MOUTH ONE (1) TO
(3) THREE INCHES FROM THE PART TO BE
ATTENDED TO, INHALE TRU THE NOSE AND
EXHALE TRU THE MOUTH, BLOWING THE
BREATH OVER THE SPOT AFECTED, AT THE
SAME TIME SINGINGING IN VERY HUSHED
WAY, (WITHOUT THE VOISE), THE WORD -
-,, YAT- HA-AH-HU-VAI-RIO-,, ,,-OM,,
VIBRATING THE,, OM,, TO THE END OF THE
BREATH. DO IT FOR FEW MINUTES, THEN
WHISPER A PRAYER TO HEAVENLY FATHER,
TO SEND THE HEALING POWER TO THE SICK
PART TO RESTORE IT TO NORMAL STATE.
ACCORDING TO THE AFFECTION, WHEN IT IS
HEATING (LOCAL HIGHER TEMPERATURE)-
- BLOW THE INCANTATIONS ON -COLD)
AND IF IT IS COOLING (LOCAL ANEMIA)
BREATH THEM ON HOT.
IF YOU CAN PUT YOUR HANDS ON, RIGHT
HAND ON THE BODY IN THE PROXIMITY
OF THE AFECTION, LEFT ON THE OPPOSITE
PART.
NOTE. (DO NOT LET THE PERSON BEING
TREATED HEAR THE WORDS, BUT CONWEY
THEM TO THE AFECTED PART, WHICH
WILL HEAR AND REACT ACCORDINGLY.

VII. ARCANE. SOUNDLESS SOUND. "AUM" VOICE OF THE SILENCE.

THIS IS HEARING OF THE VIBRATION OF THE WORLD SOUND OF RHYTM WHICH PERMEATS THE UNIVERSE THE HOLY AND SACRED "AUM".

SIT ON A CHAIR, HAVING IN FRONT OF IT A TABLE WITH A PILLOW ON IT, AT CONVENIENT HEIGHT, SO THAT YOU CAN LEAN ON IT WITH YOUR ELBOWS, WHILE HEAD RESTS ON THE PALMS OF THE HANDS EYES, FOREHEAD, AND UPPER CHEEKS RESTING ON THE PALMS OF THE HANDS WITH FOUR FINGERS OF EACH HAND, WITHOUTH THUMBS, WHICH YOU WET WITH SALIVA, AND INSERT IN THE OPENING OF THE EARS, PREVENTING THIS WAY ALL THE SOUNDS TO REACH FROM OUTSIDE KEEP YOUR SPINE STRAIGHT, BREATH DEEPLY THE TWELVE MASTER BREATHS, SEVEN (7) SECONDS INHALATION, (1) SECOND STOP (7) SEVEN SECONDS EXHALATION (1) ONE SECOND STOP (12 TIMES.). THEN RELAXED COMPLETELY, CLOSE YOUR EYES, AND LIFT THEM, (OR TURN THEM, A FAR UPWARDS AS POSSIBLE, CONVERGING THE AT THE SAME TIME, TRYING TO SEE INSIDE OF YOUR FOREHEAD BETWEEN THE EYEBROWS.

THEN FORGET EVERYTHING, AND CONCENTRATE YOUR ATTENTION ON THE 'INNER LEFT EAR, IN THE BEGINNING YOU WILL HEAR RUMBLING SOUND OF THE BLOOD, THIS WILL SUBSIDE AND YOU WILL HEAR THE SHRILL BLAST OF A TRUMPET, THEN AFTER A TIME WILL COME THE SOUND OF THE BUZZING OF A BEE, NEXT WILL BE SOUND OF THE RINGING OF A BELL, THIS GONE IN A WHILE YOU WILL HEAR THE SOUND OF A FLUTE, WHICH WILL CEASE AND, AFTER A LULL YOU WILL HEAR THE HUM OF THE RHYTM OF THE WORLD - THE SACRED "AUM". LISTEN TO IT, YOU WILL UNDERSTAND

GO IN THIS STATE TIME AND AGAIN, AND STAY IN IT AS LONG AS YOU CAN OR WANT. FIND THE TRUE SOUND OF „AUM" AND TRY TO LEARN THE SOUNDING OF IT.

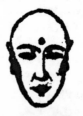

POSITION OF THE EYES. (IT IS CALLED LOOKING ON THE MOUNTAIN TOPS, TOWARD THE URNA. CENTRAL EYE BETWEEN THE EYEBROWS.

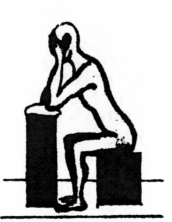

POSTURE FOR HEARING THE „AUM".

NOTE: TO GET THE BEST RESULTS, AND HAVE THEM THE QUICKEST WAY, START THE EXERCISE WITH II MASTER ARCANE. (STANDING AND TENSING EXERCISE. (FACE THE POSITION OF THE SUN.).

VII B ARCANE. CONCENTRATION.
SIT ERECT, SPINE STRAIGHT, FACING THE POSITION OF THE SUN. DO THE COMPLETE I) FIRST MASTER ARCANE (EXERCISE), THEN PROCEDE IN PRACTICE OF CONCENTRATION, - FORMULATE THE THOUGHT ON WHICH YOU WANT TO CONCENTRATE AND MAKE IT SIMPLE AND CONCRETE, THEN HOLD IT IN YOUR ATTENTION, - TURN YOUR EYES INWARD AND AS FAR UPWARD AS YOU

CAN COMFORTABLY REACH, CLOSE THEM
AS MUCH AS YOU CAN CLOSE THEM COMFOR-
TABLY. YOU WILL FIND THAT INSIDE OF
YOUR FOREHEAD, BETWEEN THE EYEBROWS
YOU FEEL A SLIGHT PRESSURE OR TENSION,
AT TIMES THE FEELING MAYBE THAT
OF SLIGHT PINCHING. HOLD TO THIS FEE-
LING, NOT LETTING IT RELAX, DO NOT
PAY ATTENTION TO YOUR BREATHING
OR YOUR BODY, (AT TIMES AFTER
EXHALATION OR IN THE MIDDLE OF
IT YOU WILL COMFORTABLY STOP
BREATHING, THIS SHOULD BE SO.)
NOW TAKE THE THOUGHT ON WHICH
YOU CONCENTRATE, TRY TO SQUISE
IT IN THE POINT BETWEEN THE
EYEBROWS WHERE YOU FEEL THE
PRESSURE. HOLD IT WITH THE PRE-
SSURE, REPEATED IN FRONT OF IT,
AND INSIDE OF IT, ON ALL THE MODES
AND MANNERS, HALF IT, SPLIT IT,
THE THOUGHT AND THE WORDS CON-
TAINED IN IT. YOU WILL KNOW THEN,
THIS IS CALLED CAREFUL OBSERVATION,
+ AT CERTAIN TIMES YOU WILL SEE LIGHT, BE-
FORE YOUR EYES, IT MAY BE A DOT, A STAR,
A EYE, A VISION OF HEAVENLY FATHER,
A GUARDIAN ANGELIC. TO SEE THOSE THINGS
PERTAINS TO SECOND STAGE OF CONCEN-
TRATION CALLED WHEN THE SUBJECT IS
OF SPIRITUAL IMPORTANCE APPEARS -
-MEDITATION. WHEN IT IS PERTAINING
TO OBJECTS OF WORLDLY LIFE IT IS THAN
CONTEMPLATION. EACH OF THOSE
HIGHEST STAGES, BEGINS WITH CONCEN-
TRATION. THE DEFINITION OF THOSE

PROCESSES IS – 1) ATTENTION , 2) RIVETING OF
ATTENTION TO THE OBJECT IS CONCENRA-
TION, IT IS ALSO CALLED SETTING THE HEART
ON THE OBJECT, 3) BECOMING AT ONE
WITH THE OBJECT IS MEDITATION OR
ACCORDING TO THE OBJECT IT MAY BE
CONTEMPLATION. (CALLED PERFORMING SANGH YAMA
DURING THE MEDITATION AND CONTEMPLA
TION ALWAYS LOOK FOR THE LIGHT, AND
IT WILL COME TO YOU, SO BRIGHT, THAT THE
LIGHT OF THE SUN WILL SEEM ONLY A
SHADOW IN COMPARISON WITH IT, IT
IS REAL, IT IS TO BE SEEN ON EVERY
PLANE – PHYSICAL, MENTAL, SPIRITUAL
AND PSYCHIC. THIS IS ILLUMINATION,
"THE LIGHT"

ALSO BEING IN PASSIVE STATE YOU WILL
SEE THE THINGS, OBJECTS, PERSONS, AND
HAPPENINGS AND EVENTS—THEN IT IS
CLAIRVOYANT STATE.
  TO HELP TO DEVELOP THIS FACULTY,
GRADUALLY GET ACCUSTOMED TO GAZE
IN THE SUN (BEFORE IT CROSSES THE
MERIDIAN), ALSO MORNINGS AND
EVENINGS, AT SUNRISE AND SUNSET,
BEGIN WITH SHORT TIME, LENGHTE-
NING IT WITH ESTABLISHING OF THE
HABIT. THE SAME TIME THAT
YOU SPEND LOOKING AT THE SUN,
USE IMMEDIATELY ON LOOKING
ON SOME DARK SPACE OR WALL,
OR CLOS YOUR EYES AND WATCH
THE SPOT THAT IS PHOTOGRAPHED
ON YOUR RETINA, TRYING TO KEEP
IT STEADY, AND WORKING TO BRINL

IT NEAR TO YOU . BETWEEN (6) SIX AND
(1) ONE FEET. YOU WILL FIND THAT
THE IMAGE SEEN BECOMES LIKE A
MIRROR FROM BURNISHED GLASS AND
METAL , IN WHICH YOU WILL SEE
REFLECTION OF YOUR FACE , AND
DIFFERENT OBJECTS AND THINGS.
    USE ALSO MOON , AND PLANETS
AND STARS, (BEFORE THEY CROSS THE
MERIDIAN)
IN THE DELOPEMENT WILL HELP TO
USE ALSO A HUNDRED WATT BLUE
ELECTRIC BULB AT 3 (THREE FEET
DISTANCE.)
USE EXERCISES TO CONTROL THE MUSCLES
OF YOUR EYES , BY ROLLING THEM OPEN
AND TIGHTLY CLOSED , BY STRIWING TO
SEE AS FAR BACK OF YOU AS YOU CAN,
AND ALSO UP AND DOWN WITHOUT MOVIN
YOUR HEAD. ROLL YOUR EYES IN DIFFE-
RENT GEOMETRICAL FIGURES. LEARN
TO CONVERGE THEM AND CROSS THEM,
LOOKING AT ,,URNA,, POINT BEETWEEN
THE EYEBROWS , AND BRINGING THEM
CROSSED TO THE TIP OF THE NOSE.
WORK TO BE ABLE TO DESRIBE GEOME-
TRICAL FIGURES WITH YOUR EYES CROSSED.
DEVELOP FACULTY OF LOOKING WITH
ONE EYE UP AND WITH ANOTHER DOWN.
    NOW COMES THE EXERCISE USED FOR
SPLITTING THE ETHER , FOR CLAIRVOYANCE
- SIT STRAIGHT, RELAXED CLOSE YOUR
 LEFT HAND LEAVING THE INDEX FINGER
OUTSTRECHED, COVER THE LEFT HAND
WITH THE SO THAT THE THREE FINGERS
OF THE RIGHT HAND WILL BE CLASPING
THE THREE FOLDED FINGERS OF THE LEFT,

69

THE FOREFINGER OF THE RIGHT HAND IS
OUTSRECHED TIP OF IT TUCHING THE FORE-
FINGER OF THE LEFT HAND, THE THUMBS
OF BOTH HANDS ARE TUCHING EACH
OTHER.
NOW SEPARATE THE FOREFINGERS OF
BOTH HANDS AND MAKE THE DISTANCE
BETWEEN THEM SAME AS THE DISTANCE
BETWEEN THE PUPILS OF THE BOTH EYES,
HOLD THE HANDS ABOUT TWO (2) FEET
FROM YOUR EYES, AND LOOK AT THE
FOREFINGERS UNTIL YOU WILL SEE
IN THE CENTER BETWEN THEM,
THE THIRD FINGER, COMPOSITE OF
TWO RORE FINGERS. (HAVING ON ITS
SIDES TWO FINGERNAILS.
STUDY THIS COMPOSITE FINGER
UNTIL YOU SEE IT PERFECTLY, AND
WHEN BECOMES TO YOU A ABSOLUTE
REALITY. MOVE YOUR HANDS FARTHER
AND NEARER TRYING TO KEEP THE
THIRD FINGER IMAGE STEADY

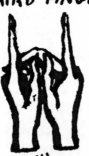

(1) POSTURE OF
THE HANDS.
(2) APPERANCE
OF THE THIRD
FINGER.

(1) (2)

LIGHT TWO CANDLES AND PUT THEM,
BETWEEN THREE AND SIX FEET AWAY,
DISTANCE BETWEEN THEM BETWEEN
3 (THREE AND FOUR INCHES, LOOK ON

70

THEM UNTIL YOU SEE THE THIRD CANDLE
BETWEEN THEM. VARY THIS EXERCISE
BY VARYING THE DISTANCE FROM THEM
AND BETWEN THEM.
   TAKE A HUMAN BEING, AND LOOK
IN THE EYES, UNTIL YOU WILL SEE THE
THIRD EYE IN BETWEEN, LEARN TO
KEEP IT STEADY WITHOUT VARYING.
   THIS GIVES THE VERY GREAT
POWER OVER HUMAN BEINGS AND
ANIMALS.
NEXT STEP IN DEVELOPING OF THE EYES
IS TO LEARN THE DISTANCE ADJUSTME-
NT AND GAIN CONSCIOUS CONTROL OVER
IT. - TAKE ANY OBJECT AND HOLD
IT NOT FAR FROM THE EYES, AFTER
THE SIGHT ADJUSTED ITSELF TO IT
REMOVE QUICKLY THE OBJECT, BUT
TRY TO KEEP THE EYES ADJUSTED
TO THE DISTANCE WHERE OBJECT
FORMERLY WAS. - THE THING
BEYOND WILL SEEM HAZY, PRAC-
CTICE UNTIL YOU CAN ADJUST YOUR
GAZE AT WILL - WATCH THE DUST
PARTICLES SUSPENDED IN THE
NEAR AIR, AND FEEL BEYOND THEM
WITHOUT CHANGING ADJUSTEMENT.
   ▪ THIS DEVELOPS THE INNER GAZE. -
NOW LOOK AT VERY FAR OBJECT, AND THEN
PUT IN THE WAY SOMETHING MUCH NEARER
WITHOUT CHANGING THE FAR SEING ADJUST-
MENT. YOU WILL PRACTICALLY LOOK THRU
THE NEAR OBJECT. PRACTICE UNTIL YOU CAN
LOOK THRU THINGS, THIS IS FAR AWAY
GAZE.

NOW YOU CAN DO CRYSTAL GAZING. FOR
CLAIRVOYANCE AND ALSO TO TRANMU-
TE THE THOUGHTS AT A DISTANCE.
  SIT ON THE CHAIR, RELAX, DO THE FIRST
MASTER ARCANE' (EXRCISE), THAN HAVE
IN FRONT OF YOU A TABLE ON WHICH YOU
CAN REST YOUR ELBOWS. - REST UPPER
PART OF YOUR FACE ON THE PALMS
AND FINGERS, BUT THUMBS PLACE
BEHIND THE EARS. HAVE THE BALL
OF CRYSTAL, ON A STAND LITTE HIGHER
THAT LEVEL OF YOUR EYES. (YOU CAN
USE, GLASS BALL, TOURMALINE, BERYL,
MAGICAL MIRROR, OR GLASS BALL FIL-
LED WITH WATER, ALSO FIRE.)
HAVE A SINGLE CANDLE BURNING UP
BEHIND YOU, WHILE IN FRONT OF
YOU, BEHIND THE CRYSTAL HAVE A
DARK SCREEN PREFERABLY BLACK
VELVET.
  PROCEDE TO GAZE AND CONCENTRATE
IN THE CRYSTAL, SPLITTING LIGHTLY
THE ETHER UNTIL YOU WILL SEE TWO
REFLECTIONS OF THE CANDLE.
WATCH PATIENTLY, THE THINGS WILL
BEGIN TO APPEAR, AND GET CLEAR.
PRACTICE ALWAYS EVERY DAY AT THE
SAME TIME WITHIN THE HOUR.
TIME - FROM 5 (FIVE) TO 30 (THIRTY) MI-
NUTES WITHOUT BLINKING. (FOLLOW THE SUN)
YOU CAN DO ALSO WATCHING FORMS
HOLDING YOUR HAND (RIGHT) OVVER YOUR
FACE AND PRESSING SLIGHTLY ON THE
TOP OF THE BRIDGE OF THE NOSE, WITH
THE EYES CLOSED. THEN YOU SEE

72

THING OUTLINED ON THE DARK SCREEN,
VERY OFTEN SYMBOLIC. THIS BRANCH
IS VERY GOOD IN READING THOUGHT FORM,
        IN NICE WARM WEATHER LAY DOWN
ON YOUR SPINE ON THE GRASS, OR SAND,
OR EARTH AND PUT YOUR ARMS FOLDING
THEM BEHIND YOUR NECK AND HEAD AS
A PILLOW, AND WATCH THE BLUE SKY
TRYING TO PENETRATE AS FAR AS POSSI-
BLE, - DO IT ALSO AT NIGHT TRYING TO
REACH THE STARS. - THIS MAKES EYES
SENSITIVE TO ULTRAVIOLET AND INFRA-
RED RAYS AND DEVELOPES FACULTY
OF SEING AURA, OF HUMANS AND
OTHER BEINGS. (ALSO PSYCHING OBJECTS,)
THIS GIVES THE WAYS OF CONCENTRATION,
MEDITATION, CONTEMPLATION, SPLITTING
OF THE ETHER, INWARD SIGHT, FARAWAY
GASE, CLAIRVOYANCE, THOUGHT FORM REA-
DING, AURA, AND PSYCHOMETRY.
X) FOR TELEPATHIC TRANSFERENCE, USE
  SAME MEANS LIKE CRYSTAL GAZING, ONLY
INSTEAD OF BEIN RECEPTIVE (PASSIVE,
BLANK) REPEAT THE FORMULA YOU WANT
TO CONVEY TO OTHER PERSON, AND
TUNE ON ACTIVE STATE (WILL POWER,
AND DESIRE.).

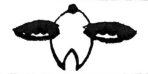

VIII G ARCANE. DREAM CONSCIOUSNESS

THE FIRST (1) STATE OF CONSCIOUSNESS IS
THE [IGNORANT STATE], SECOND (2) IS
THE [PHYSICAL STATE], THIRD IS THE
DREAM STATE, WHEN ONE IS FULLY
AWAKE OUTSIDE OF THE BODY, DURING

73

THE SLEEP, BEING CONSCIOUS, ONE CAN MOVE
AROUND IN THE ASTRAL BODY, LEARN THINGS,
BE ABLE TO PERFOM THINGS, TRU REACHING
STATE CALLED [OCCULT STATE OF CONSCIOUSNESS,
AND OTHER STATES. I.E - MENTAL, SPIRITUAL,
ASTRAL, SUPER, SELF AND COSMIC STATES OF
CONSCIOUSNESS.
TO REACH AWAKENING IN YOUR DREAM,
YOU MUST SET ASIDE A DAY COMPLETELY
TO YOURSELF, IN A PLACE FRE FROM THE
OUTSIDE DISTUBANCES.
THEN PROCEDE WITH THE WORK, BY SITTING
ON A CHAIR HAVING IN FRONT OF YOU A TABLE
WITH A PILLOW ON IT, BEND TOWARD THE
TABLE SO THAT YOU CAN PUT YOUR ELBOWS ON
IT, KEEPING THE SPINE STRAIT, REST UPPER
PART OF YOUR FACE AND FOREHEAD ON PALMS
OF YOUR HANDS WITH FINGER LITTLE SPREAD,
WET YOUR THUMBS AND INSERT THEM INTO
EARS. CLOSE YOUR EYES AND TURN THEM
SLIGHTLY UPWARD. (POSTURE EXACTLY LIKE
THE (6) SIXT L. ARCANE - SOUNDLESS SOUND
"AUM"). NOW BEGIN TO SING A MANTRA IN A
LOW VOICE - " HUONG, YANG, YANG, YANG, -
HUONG, YANG, ▮ YANG " - HUONG, YANG YANG,
YANG - HOUNG, YANG, YANG " REPEATING IT
INCESSANTLY ON A MANTRAM TUNE .

PROCEED SINGING THE MANTRAM WITHOUT
VARIATIONS FOR TWO HOURS: (WITH EARS

STOPPED.). THEN STOP THE PRACTICE AND REST
FOR TWO HOURS. IF YOU ARE HUNGRY TAKE
SOME SOLID FOOD, ABSOLUTELY RESTRAINING
ALL DAY FROM WATER, LIQUIDS AND LI-
QUID FOOD. AFTER REST OF TWO HOURS,
BEGIN AGAIN THE SAME PRACTICE AS
BEFORE SINGING THE SAME MANTRAM,
FOR TWO HOURS. AGAIN TWO HOURS REST
AND AGAIN TWO HOURS PRACTICE.
THE EXERCISE SHOULD BE DONE THREE
TIMES OF TWO HOURS EACH,
AFTER THE LAST EXERCISE, REST AND GO TO
SLEEP. IN THE BEGINNING WILL BE HARD TO
FALL TO SLEEP, BUT IT WILL COME, AND
DURING THE SLEEP YOU WILL HEAR THE
MANTRAM WHICH YOU SANG DURING THE
EXERCISES. -
NOW YOU HAVE TO WAIT A WEEK WITH
THE SECOND PART OF THE WORK, AND
AGAIN SET A DAY ASIDE.
THEN PROCEDE WITH THE EXERCISE EXAC-
TLY LIKE THE PRECEDING. ONLY NOW
USE ANOTHER MANTRAM AND ANOTHER
TUNE. (THE EARS STOPPED) IN A LOW VOICE. -

SING IT FOR TWO HOURS STRAIGHT, AND REST
FOR TWO HOURS. (THIS DAY YOU CAN DRINK
WATER, BUT CAN NOT EAT ALL DAY ABSOLUTELY

RESTRAINING FROM FOOD, THEN AGAIN REPEAT
THE SAME EXERCISES AND REST UNTIL YOU DONE
THREE EXERCISES OF TWO HOURS EACH.
REST AND GO TO SLEEP.
DURING THE SLEEP YOU WILL HEAR THE
MANTRAM YOU HAVE BEEN SINGING THIS
DAY.
THEN THE MANTRAM THAT YOU HAVE BEEN
SINGING WEEK AGO, WILL OCCUR TO YOU,
YOU WILL RECOGNISE IT, AND SUDDENLY
UNDERSTAND AND REMEMBER THAT IT IS
A MANTRAM THAT YOU HAVE BEEN SIN-
GING A WEEK AGO, WHILE THE OTHER
ONE IS THE MANTRAM YOU WERE SIN-
GING THE PREVIOUS DAY. THIS OCCURENCE
WILL GIVE ORIENTATION IN YOUR ACTIONS,
BRINGING YOU THE FULFILMENT OF THE
TASK THAT YOU UNDERTOOK, CONSCIOUS-
NESS IN YOUR DREAMING STATE.
   THE POSTURE, LACK OF FOOD, OR DRINK TOGE-
THER WITH VIBRATIONS OF SINGING THE MAN-
TRAS, IMPRESSES THE SUBCONSCIOUS AND
THE SOUL, BRINGING IN REALISATION OF
DREAM CONSCIOUSNESS.
NOTE. DURING THE EXERCISES FACE THE DI-
RECTION OF THE SUN. BE RELAXED AND
COMFORTABLE.
   ALSO ████████ REMEMBER SLEEP
ALWAYS WITH THE HEAD TOWARD NORTH,
(IN THE NIGHT TIME) IT PERMITS THE MAG-
NETIC AND ELECTRIC CURRENTS OF THE BODY,
GET STRENGHTENED WITH THE MAGNETIC
FIELDS OF THE EARTH, AND ELECTRIC CUR-
RENTS OF THE SUN. ALSO WATCH YOUR POS-

TURES WHEN FALLING TO SLEEP, IF YOU NEED
ENERGY ON PHYSICAL AND SPIRITUAL PLANES
LAY ON YOUR LEFTSIDE, ESTABLISHING
SUN BREATH, AND POSITIVENESS, — WHEN
YOU NEED ENERGY FOR STUDY OR PEACEFULL
ENDEAVORS, FALL TO SLEEP ON YOUR RIGHT
SIDE ESTABLISHING MOON BREATH, AND
PASSIVENESS — INTELLECTUAL AND PSYCHIC
PLANES, TRY ALWAYS TO BALANCE THE
NUMBER OF POSITIVE AND PASSIVE ATTITU-
DES.
WHEN NOT WELL TRY TO GIVE SHOCK
TO YOUR ENERGIES CHANGING YOUR
DIRECTION FROM NORTH TO SOUTH, WHEN
YOU GO TO SLEEP.

WHEN CONSCIOUS IN YOUR SLEEP, USE PRINCI-
PLES OF — CAREFUL OBSERVATION, CORRECT
INTERPRETATION AND PRACTICAL APPLI-
CATION. — IN THE END OF YOUR SLEEP
THE SILVER CORD WILL GUIDE YOU BACK TO
YOUR ABODE OF FLESH.
CONSCIOUS IN YOUR DREAM ACT ACCORDING
TO „— YAT-HA-AH-HU-VAI-RIO " —
„THE WILL OF THE LORD IS THE LAW OF RIGHT
EUSNESS "

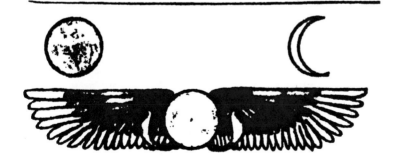

XL. ARCANE. RECHARGING NERVOUS ENERGY

A WAY USED IN ANCIENT EGYPT FOR STRENG-
HTENING OF CURRENTS OF ENERGY WITHIN
THE BODY. IT WAS SHOWN IN THE FIGURES,
USING THE SECOND MASTER ARCANE EXER-
CISE. TWO RODS CLASPED IN THE HANDS
OF STANDING FIGURES, WERE *THE GRIPS*
OF *TREMENDOUS POWER*, A KIN TO ELECT-
RICITY (SECONDARY ELECTRICITY), WHICH WHEN
THE GRIPS WERE HELD IN THE HANDS RELEA-
SED THIS ENERGY INTO THE BODY, TO BE
STORED IN UNIPOLAR GANGLIAS, AND SPINAL
FLUID, RAISING THE POTENTIAL OF ENERGY
ONE HUNDRED PERCENT, AND LASTING
FOR A DAY AND A NIGHT, (24) TWENTY FOUR
HOURS.
THE RODS WERE TWO IN NUMBER AND OF
DIFFERENT COMPOSITIONS. ONE GENERALLY
TO BE USED IN THE RIGHT, ANOTHER IN THE
LEFT HAND. ONE HAVING THE POWER OF THE
SUN, ANOTHER OF THE MOON.
THE SUN ROD OF POWER IS COMPOSED OF HARD
COAL SPECIALLY HARDENED, IN WHICH STUC-
TURE OF THE MOLECULES IS CHANGED THE
WAY THE MOLECULES OF IRON ARE CHANGED
WHEN CONVERTING IRON INTO MAGNESS.
(TO CONVERT IRON INTO MAGNESS, THE
STRUCTURE OF IRON MOLECULES IS CHAN-
GED BY RECRYSTALLISATION PROCESS —
— HARDENING, THEN IT WILL RETAIN
THE MAGNETISM) — PROCESS OF HARDENING
IS HEATING TO HIGH TEMPERATURE AND THEN
INSTANTLY COOLING BY SUBMERGING IN WA-
TER. (THE RODS OF HARD COAL PREPARED FOR
THE ELECTRIC ARC LAMPS, ARE EXELENT
AS SUN RODS OF POWER.

THE HARDENED ROD OF COAL, CAN BE INSER-
TED IN A COPPER TUBE, WITH BOTH ENDS
OPEN OR CLOSED. (LENGHT OF ROD (6") SIX
INCHES, DIAMETER (1" ONE INCH), OR
ACCORDING TO THE GRIP OF THE HAND.

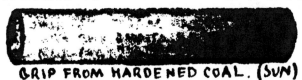

GRIP FROM HARDENED COAL. (SUN)

THE MOON ROD OF POWER IS COMPOSED OF
HARD LODE STONE, OR PRESSED LODE STONE.
(IT MAYBE ALSO A ROD OF MAGNETISED HARD
IRON OR STEEL (MAGNESS)). MOON ROD OF
POWER CAN BE INSERTED IN A ZINC, OR
TIN, TUBE, WITH BOTH ENDS OPEN OR CLO-
SED. (LENGHT AND DIAMETER IDENTICAL
WITH SUN ROD)

GRIP FROM HARDENED LODE STONE. (MOON)
THE MOON GRIP, (ROD) WORKS AS A KIND OF CATA-
LYST, TO BRING THE SUN GRIP (ROD) INTO MORE
POWERFUL ACTION.
  GRIPS AND RODS OF POWER, WERE KNOWN AND
USED IN THE MOST REMOTE EVEN TIMES, AND
  SECRETS OF PREPARATION OF THEM WAS
KNOWN TO FEW INITIATES.
THE MYSTERIOUS METAL (BRONZE) AURI-
CALLUM HAS TREMENDOUS POWER, AND
IS COMPOSED OF FIVE METALS, EACH HA-
VING A DEFINITE COLOR - WHITE, BLACK,
RED, BLUE AND YELLOW. IT IS RADIOACTIVE,
AND IN IT HIDES MYSTERY OF IMACULATE

CONCEPTION. (PROPORTION OF METALS IS EVEN).
THEN COMES ELECTRON, COMPOSED OF GOLD
AND SILVER (40% GOLD AND 60% SILVER),
THEN COMBINATION OF SILVER 75% AND ZINC 25%
; COMBINATION OF COPPER AND ZINC, AND ALSO
COPPER AND TIN. (MANY COMBINATIONS
OF BRONZE YOU CAN MAKE FIGURING OUT
PLANETS THEIR RELATIONS AND PROPERTIES.
SUN ☉-GOLD, MOON ☾-SILVER, SATURN ♄-LEAD
JUPITER ♃-TIN, MARS ♂-IRON, VENUS ♀-COPPER
MERCURY ☿-MERCURY.
ALSO MINERALS — COAL, LODESTONE, BERYL, AMBER,
TOURMALINE, ROCK CRYSTAL, HEMATITE, ETC.

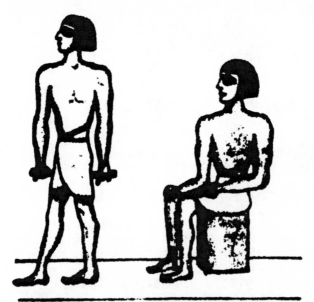

THE EGYPTIAN MASTER SYSTEM POSTURES FOR RE-
CHARGING THE NERVOUS ENERGY. (ONE SHOULD BE
RELAXED, AND FOLLOWING THE DIRECTION OF THE
SUN.)

OBJECTS SHAPED IN DIFFENT SYMBOLIC FORMS ARE
ALSO USED TROUGHOVT THE WORLD, LIKE BABYLO-
NIAN MACES (IRON WITH SILVER INLAY) WITH
HORNED HUMAN HEAD, AND HEAD OF THE
BULL.) IN THIBET IS USED DORGEE, ETC.
RODS OF POWER CAN BE USED WITH SECOND ARCANE

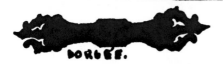

DORGEE.

X L.ARCANE. KECHARA MUDRA. (POSTURE)
IT IS USED, FOR PREPATION FOR HIBERNATING,
(GOING INTO LETARGIC TRANCE), AND
ALSO ENABLES ONE TO CENTER THE LIFE
ENERGIES IN THE HEAD, SEPARATING THE
POLES IN THE BODY, BY CLOSING BOTH
CURRENTS INDIVIOVALLY, BY WHICH MEANS
THEY MAY REMAIN FOR INDEFINTE
TIME, BUT IN REALITY - 3 TO 6 MONTHS
IS USED. -
KECHARA MUDRA IS PROCESS OF SWALLO-
WING THE TONGUE OR OF INSERTING THE
TONGUE PAST SOFT PALATE INTO NASAL
CAVITIES.
IT SHOULD BE PREPARED SLOWLY AND
PRACTISED GRADVALLY.
EVERY DAY, YOU MUST FOR CERTAIN TIME
STICK OUT YOUR TONGUE, GET HOLD OF
IT WITH YOUR HAND TROUGH A PIECE OF
CLOTH (TO PREVENT THE TONGUE FROM
SLIPPING FROM THE FINGERS.), THEN
PULL THE TONGUE OUT, GRADVALLY

MAKING IT LONGER, YOU MUST PULL IT, AND
ALSO MASSAGE IT WITH A MILKING MOTION.
DURING PULLING OF THE TONGUE, THE MEM-
BRANE UNDER THE TONGUE, CALLED, FRŒNU-
LUM LINGUDE,, WILL BECOM LOOSENED OR
CUT ON THE ▬▬▬ TEETH, PERMITTING THE
TONGUE TO GRADUALLY BECOME LONGER.
(CUTTING OF THE, FRŒNULUM LINGUDE, MAY
BE DONE BY OPERATION, KNIFE, OR USING
A SHARP BLADE OF GRASS.) ALWAYS AFTER
INJURING THE TONGUE TROUGH PULLING APPLY THE
SALT TO THE WOUND. REAL PERFECTION IS REACHED
WHEN ONE CA TOUCH WITH THE TONGUE, POINT
BETWEEN THE EYEBROWS.

XI L. ARCANE. MULLAH MUDRA. MULLHA MUDRA
USED IN THE DEVELOPEMENT FOR HIBERNATION,
ALSO FOR REJUVENATION AND CLEANING OF
THE INTESTINAL TRACT AND LOWER BOWEL,
IT IS VERY HEALING IN CASE OF GASTRITIS, AND
APPENDIX.
FACE THE SUN, (OR THE DIRECTION OF), GO DOWN
ON YOUR KNEES, STRAIGTEN THE SPINE WITH
ARMS AND HANDS UP, LOOKING SLIGHTLY UPWA
RDS. RELAX, DRAW THE BREATH IN STRONGLY
AND FULLY, BENDING SLIGHTLY (SWAYING) BACK-
WARDS, THEN HOLDING THE BREATH, BEND
FORWARD UNTIL YOU CAN BEND THE THE ARMS
AT THE ELBOWS, AND REST YOUR ELBOWS AND
FOREARMS ON THE EARTH, THEN SWING ON
ELBOWS AND KNEES, (UPPER ARMS AND TIGHS)
SO THAT YOU CAN COMFORTABLY TOUCH THE
GROUND WITH YOUR FOREHEAD. (THIS IS CALLED
PROSTRATING ONE SELF). ELBOWS SHOULD BE FROM
12" TO 24" FROM THE KNEES). RELEASE THE BREATH THE
MOMENT YOU STRIKE THE EARTH WITH THE ELBOWS.
RELAX. TAKE A PREVIOUSLY PREPARED LITTLE TUBE.
- FROM BAMBOO, HARD RUBBER, WOOD, IVORY, OR
OTHER APPROPRIATE SUBSTANCE, (ABOUT 5" TO 6"
LONG, 1/2" WIDE (DIAMETER), OPENING INSIDE THE TUBE
1/8 TO 1/4", ENDS VERY WELL ROUNDED AND POLISHED
THE TUBE YOU MUST INSERT INTO ANUS, PAST
EXTERNAL AND INTERNAL SPHINCTERS, WHICH

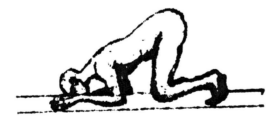

83

WILL BE ABOUT 3" (THREE INCHES), AT THE CORRECT
INSERTION OF THE TUBE, THE PASSAGE FOR AIR
WILL BE ESTABLISHED, AND YOU WILL HEAR A
SPECIFIC HISSING SOUND, OF AIR PASSING TO
AND FROM THE LARGE INTESTINE.
TO REGULATE IT ADJUST YOUR POSTURE SWAY-
ING FORWARD AND BACKWARD, ON YOUR
ELBOWS AND KNEES. KEEP YOUR STOMACH
RELAXED, AND BREATH EVENLY AND RHYT-
MICALLY, USING MOSTLY CHEST MUSCLES,
IN DEEP INHALATIONS AND EXHALATIONS,
YOU WILL NOTICE THAT DURING THE INHALA-
TION, THE AIR IS EXPELLED FROM THE IN-
TESTINES, AND DURING THE EXHALATION
THE AIR IS BEING DRAWN IN THRU THE RECTUM
THIS IS CALLED MULLAH MUDRA, BREA-
THING TROUGH THE RECTUM. OCCASIONALLY
YOU CAN CLOSE YOUR LARYNX AND PERFORM
MUSCULAR ACT OF BREATHING, WITHOUT CIRCU-
LATING THE AIR IN THE LUNGS. THIS STREA-
GHTENS THE INTESTINES, AND MAKES AWAY
WITH THE INDIGESTIONS AND CONSTIPATION.

FORM OF TUBE USED WITH THIS EXERCISE
(NOTE! TUBE MAY BE ALSO SLIGHTLY BENT.]
DO THIS EXERCISE BETWEEN 10.- (TEN) AND
30 (THIRTY) MINUTES. OR ACCORDING TO NEED
   OCCASIONALLY DURING THE EXERCISE FOR
MORE COMFORT YOU CAN MOVE THE HANDS
NEAR EACH OTHER AND REST YOUR FOREHEAD
OR FACE ON KNUCKLES OF YOUR HANDS.
   ALSO ACCORDING TO FELT NEED YOU MAY
RAISE UPRIGHT ON YOUR KNEES, AND PUT

YOUR ARMS AND HANDS UP, BENDING BACK
WARD, LIKE IN THE BEGINNING OF EXERCI
SE, INHALING DEEPLY.
REMEMBER ALWAYS AT THE END OF
THE EXERCISE TAKE CARE, THAT THE
AIR IS EXPELLED, WHAT MEANS YOU TAKE
THE DEEP INHALATION, AND REMOVE THE TUBE
FROM THE RECTUM WHILE HOLDING BREATH
A PUSHING IT DOWNWARD, (TENSING)
NOTE |THE TUBE SHOULD BE KEPT CLEAN.

X X X

XII) G.S. ARCANE. FACE AND HEAD REJUVE-
NATING EXERCISE. ALSO GENERAL.
THIS IS THE EXERCISE WHICH IS ACTUALLY A COMPLI
MENTORY TO THE XITH ARCANE (MULLAH, OR MULLHA
MUDRA, AND IS USED TO REJUVENATE AND CLEAN
THE FACE, NECK, HEAD, AND ALSO TO REFRESH
REJUVENATE AND STRENGHTEN THE ORGANS
IN THE HEAD. -BRAIN, ORGANS OF HEARING
TASTE, SMELL, SINUSES, E.T.C. GETTING AWAY
WITH ALL THE CONGESTIONS, STASIS, AND UN-
HEALTHY CONDITIONS, WITHIN BOUNDARIES
OF THE HEAD, HAIR AND TEETH INCLUDED.
THE OUTSIDE OF THE HEAD AND FACE, CAN BE AFFE
CTED BY WASHING WITH WATER, CREAMS, LOTIONS
HOT AND COLD APPLICATIONS, MASSAGE ETC.,
BUT THOSE THINGS IN TIME DO MORE DAMAGE
THAN HELP BY STRETCHING AND DEFORMING
THE CELLS, WHICH LOOSE THEIR ELASTICITY
AND THUS BECOME LIFELESS AND FLABBY.

85

EVERY BODY IS CONSISTING OF CELLS, THE UNIT OF
PROTOPLASMIC MASS IS A CELL, HAVING A CELL
BODY, CELL-WALL, CELL-NUCLEUS AND NUCLEO-
LUS, AS IT'S TYPICAL AND FUNDAMENTAL CHARACTE
RS. ATTRACTION-SPHERE ENCLOSING
TWO CENTROSOMES

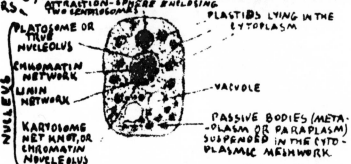

PLATOSOME OR TRUE NUCLEOLUS

CHROMATIN NETWORK

LININ NETWORK

NUCLEUS

KARYOSOME NET KNOT, OR CHROMATIN NUCLEOLUS

PLASTIDS LYING IN THE CYTOPLASM

VACUOLE

PASSIVE BODIES (META-
-PLASM OR PARAPLASM)
SUSPENDED IN THE CYTO-
PLASMIC MESHWORK

PROTOPLASM CONSISTS OF COMPOUND OF CARBON
(OVER 50%), HYDROGEN, NITROGEN, OXYGEN,
SMALL AMOUNT OF SULPHUR, PHOSPHORUS, AND
ABOUT A DOSEN OTHER ELEMENTS.
CELLS ARE OF MANY KINDS, BUT FUNDAMENTA-
LLY THEY ARE ALL SIMILAR IN CONSTITUTION
AND POWERS. ALL LIVING BODIES CONSIST OF ONE
OR MORE PROTOPLASMIC CELLS AND CERTAIN EXTRA-
PROTOPLASMIC ELEMENTS, PRODUCTS OF CELLULAR
ACTIVITY.
ONE OF THE MOST REMARKABLE OF THE CHARAC-
TERS OF LIVING THINGS IS THEIR POWER TO
TAKE UP NON-LIVING MATTER, CONVERT IT
INTO LIVING SUBSTANCE AND BACK AGAIN
INTO LIFELESS MATTER, A PROCESS CALLED
NUTRITION. THE FIRST PART OF THIS PRO-
CESS, THAT BY WHICH THE NON-LIVING
MATTER BECOMES LIVING, IS CALLED
ANABOLISM. THE REVERSE PROCESS,
WHICH RETURNS LIVING MATTER TO THE
LIFELESS STATE, IS CATABOLISM.

ANABOLISM IS THE PROCESS BY WHICH INERT
FOOD SUBSTANCES, SIMPLE COMPOUNDS, ARE
BUILT UP INTO COMPLEX SPECIAL COMPOUNDS
MANFESTING THE PROPERTIES OF LIFE.
CATABOLISM IS THE PROCESS BY WHICH
THE COMPLEX, LIVING COMPOUNDS ARE
RETURNED TO A MORE SIMPLE FORM BY
A PROCESS OF COMBUSTION, CHEMICALLY
SIMILAR TO BURNING, ALWAYS PRODUCING
CARBON DIOXIDE (CO_2) AND WATER AND IN
MANY CASES VARIOUS FORMS OF ASH.
ANABOLIC PROCESS SUPPLIES THE MATERIAL
FOR CATABOLISM AND IN EXCESS OF THIS NEED
GIVES GROWTH, OR INCREASE OF TISSUE.
THE CATABOLIC PROCESS YIELDS ENERGY IN
THE BODY.
THE METABOLIC PROCESS IS CHARACTERISED BY
THE CONSUMPTION OF OXYGEN (O) AND THE EVO-
LUTION OF CARBON DIOXIDE (CO_2). THIS PROCESS
IS CALLED RESPIRATION.
OXYGEN SUPPLIES THE ELEMENT NECESSARY,
FOR THE COMBUSTION OF FOOD AND TISSUE
SUBSTANCES AND IS NECESSARY IN THE CA-
TABOLIC PHASE OF METABOLISM. IT SUP-
PORTS THE DESTRUCTIVE PROCESS AND DOES
NOT ENTER THE PRODUCTIVE, ANABOLIC PROCESS
EXEPT AS SOME DEGREE OF ENERGY IS CONSU-
MED IN BUILDING THE LIFELESS MATERIALS
INTO LIVING SUBSTANCE. HOWEVER SOME
OXYGEN IS STORED IN THE TISSUES WHERE
IT REMAINS INERT UNTIL NEEDED FOR
COMBUSTION FOR THE PRODUCTION OF ENER-
GY. CONSIDERABLE PERCENTAGE OF OXYGEN
IS ALWAYS A PART OF PROTOPLASM ITSELF
 NEXT TO OXYGEN, LIVING THINGS NEED
WATER (H_2O). THE SIMPLEST FORMS OF LIFE,
AND MANY OTHERS LIVE ENTIRELY IN WA-
TER. WATER MAKES UP THE LARGER
PART OF ALL LIVING THINGS.

IN ADDITION TO THE WATER INCORPORATED
INTO THE CELLS AS A PART OF THEIR TISS-
UES, ALL THE ACTIVE, LIVING CELLS OF THE
MANY-CELLED BEINGS LIVE IN A WHAT
HAS TO BE CONSIDERED FLUID MEDIUM,
MAIN CONTINUENT OF WHICH IS WATER.
IN CASE OF THE PLANTS THIS ▬▬▬▬
FLUID IS CALLED SAP; IN THE ANIMALS
AND MAN IT IS BLOOD OR LYMPH,
OR JUST WATER WHICH IS CIRCULATED
TO THE TISSUES, THOSE BODY FLUIDS CONVEY
TO THE CELLS THEIR FOOD, CARRY AVAY THEIR
WASTES, AND SUPPLY THE WATER NECESSARY
FOR KEEPING THE LIVING SUBSTANCE IN THE
HALF-FLUID, MOBILE CONDITIONS NECESSARY
TO LIFE.
WHEN THERE IS INSUFICIENT SUPPLY OF FLUID
MEDIUM, BLOOD OR LYMPH, TO THE CELLS,
IT AFFECTS THEM BY NOT FEEDING THEM, AND
THEY BECOME UNDERNURISHED AND STARWED,
AND ALSO THE ELIMINATION AND COMBUS-
TION PROCESS BECOMES SLOW, LEAVING
LOTS OF WASTES WITHIN THE CELLS, NOT ELIM-
NATED, WHICH CLOGG THE CELLS ADDING UNNECE-
SSARY BULK, STRETCHING THEIR PROTECTIVE
MEMBRANE AND TAKING AWAY ITS ELASTICITY.

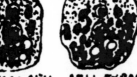

IN THE CASE OF BAD
METABOLISM, THE WALLS
OF THE CELL WILL BE EX-
PANDED, BUT LIQUID
CONTENT WILL BE SMA-
LLER, EXPANSION DUE TO
REFUSE COLLECTED.

NORMAL CELL   CELL EXPANDED
TRU BADMETABO-
LISM.

CELLS NOT POSSESSING ELASTICITY AND LIQUI-
DITY, FIT BADLY TOGETHER, AND TEND TO STAY
IN THE FORM FORCED ON THEM WITH MO-
VEMENTS OF THE PARTS OF THE BODY, OR

ORGANS, WITHOUT HAVING ENOUGH SPRINGI
NESS TO RETURN TO NORMAL SUSPENTION-
-TENTION. THIS CREATES WRINKLES AND
FOLDS, OBSTRUCTING EVEN MORE PROCE-
SSES OF METABOLISM, AND CREATES GRA-
DUALLY DEPOSITS OF SALTS, IN CAPPILA-
RIES, AND TISSUES AND ARTERIES AND
VEINS, BRINGING A STATE CALLED –
HARDENING OF THE ARTERIES –ARTE-
RIO SCLEROSIS.
THE ARTERIES RESPONDING TO ADRENALIN
AND EPHEDRINE OFTEN RELEASED IN THEM
FROM THE ADRENALS, CALLED FORTH BY
HIGH TENSION OF LIVING, CONTRACT-AND
GET SALTS DEPOSITED IN THEM, HARDENING
MORE AND BRINGING THE HIGH BLOOD
PRESSURE, AND GENERAL DEBILITY.
   THE ONLY MEDICINE FOR THIS STATE,
IS TO RESTORE THE DISOLVING AND CU-
RING TONE OF THE BLOOD, AND THEN
TO DIRECT IT TOWARD UNDERNURISHED
AND CONGESTED WITH REFUSE AREAS,
THRU CONSCIOUS APPLICATION OF
THIS ARCANE.
1ST PART – PURIFYING AND STRENGH-
TENING OF THE BLOOD.
DRINK PLENTY WATER, FRUIT AND VEGE-
TABLE JUICES – [LEMONS, ORANGES, PINE-
APPES, PRUNES, APPLES, ETC. –
CELERY, ONIONS, CARROTS, BEETS, CABBA-
GES ETC.
DRINK MILK ONE HOUR OR MORE AFTER
TAKING JUICES, AFTER MILK YOU CAN
TAKE JUICES TWO HOURS OR AFTER.
USE XI ARCANE MULLAH (MULLHA) MUDRA.
IF YOU HAVE TO MAKE THE REJUVENATION
STRONGER, USE JUICES OF BEETS, CELERY,
CARROTS, ORANGES AND TURNIPS, AND AFTER

89

HEATING THEM LITTLE BELOW BODY TEMPERA
TURE, DILUTED IN 50% WATER (TOGETHER
1 QUART) USE AS ENEMA EVERY THREE DAYS.
AS TO REGULAR FOOD, EAT EVERYTHING YOU
LIKE, OR ARE USED TO, BUT IN SMALLER
QUANTITIES (ON ACCOUNT OF JUICES AND
MILK THAT YOU ARE TAKING.

NOW COMES THE EXERCISE TO BE DONE
TWICE EVERY DAY, FOR A PERIOD FROM
5 (FIVE) TO 10 (TEN) MINUTES. THIS EXER-
CISE IS MADE TO AWAKEN AND INTENSIFY
WORK OF THYROID AND PAPATHYROID GLAND
WHICH, RELEASE SECRETIONS, TO STRENGHTEN'
AND PURIFY THE BLOOD, AND HEIGHTEN THE META-
BOLISM, HELPING TO DISSOLVE AND ELIMINATE SALTS
AND VASTE PRODUCTS FROM THE BODY.

1) PUT YOUR THUMB FIRMLY UNDER THE CHIN,
OTHER FINGERS FOLDED. PRESS SLIGHTLY
WITH THE TUMB ON THE MUSCLES UNDER THE
CHIN. NOW ROLL YOUR TONGUE BACKWARDS
AND FORWARD, REPEATING THIS MOTIONS
FOR 2½ TO 5 MINUTES. (YOU WILL FEEL THE
MUSCLES RIPPLE UNDER YOUR CHIN, WHERE
YOUR THUMB RESTS, HELP THIS MOTION
FOLLOWING IT WITH THE THUMB, SLIGHTLY
PRESSING TO EXCITE THE CONTRACTION OF THE
MUSCLES.) THIS IS THE FIRST PART OF THE
EXERCISE.

2) BEND YOUR HEAD DOWN UNTIL CHIN WILL
TOUCH THE CHEST, THEN TENSE THE MUSCLES
OF THE CHIN AND NECK, BY STRETCHING
THE MOUTH ON BOTH SIDES AND DOWN.
ALL THE MUSCLES AND TENDONS SHOULD
STAND OUT ON THE NECK, PROCEDE THEN
TO LIFT THE HEAD AND THE CHIN WAY UP
WITHOUT RELEASING THE TENTION OF'

THE MUSCLES, BUT INSTEAD PULLING THEM
AND STRETCHING VIGOROUSLY.
AFTER PULLING THE CHIN AND THE HEAD
WAY UP, RELAX THE NECK AND FACE,
BEND THE HEAD AND CHIN DOWN AGAIN,
TENSE AND REPEAT THE BEFORE DESCRI-
BED EXERCISE. DO IT REPEATING FOR
2 1/2 TO 5 MINUTES.-
THOSE TWO ABOVE DESCRIBED EXERCISES,
AWAKEN, PURIFY AND EXCITE THE THYROID
GLAND, WHICH PRODUCES AND SEND INTO
THE BLOOD STREAM, SECRETIONS WHICH
ARE REJUVENATING TO THE TISSUES AND
THE BODY.
NOTE: IN THE BEGINNING OF THOSE
EXERCISES YOU WILL HAVE PAINS IN
THE THROAT, NECK AND THYROID AREA,
WHICH IS PERFECTLY TO BE EXPECTED,
ON ACCOUNT OF EXERCISING THE MUSCLES,
WHICH ARE NOT USED TO GYMNASTIC.
AFTER FEW DAYS THE PAINS WILL STOP
AS YOU ATTAIN THE CONTROL OVER THE
MUSCLES, BEST BEGIN WITH 2 1/2 MINU-
TES EACH EXERCISE AND GRADUALLY
BUILD UP TO 5 MINUTES
WE COME NOW TO THE PROPER XII ARCANE
REJUVENATING FACE AND HEAD. IT IS AS FAR
AS THE POSTURE GOES IDENTICAL WITH MULLAN
(MULLHA) MUDRA, WITHOUT USING BREATHING
TROUGH THE RECTUM, AND RAISING MORE
OFTE TO THE UPRIGHT POSITION ON YOUR
KNEES.- DO VERY STRONG AND DEEP
BREATHING, FOR ABOUT FIVE MINUTES,
UNTIL YOUR FACE AND BODY WILL START
TINGLING, SHOWING STRONG OXYDISATION
OF THE BLOOD. THEN FACING THE DIRECTION

OF THE SUN GO DOWN ON YOUR KNEES, STRAIGH
TEN THE SPINE WITH ARMS AND HAND EXTEN-
DED UPWARDS, POINTING THE EYES SLIGHTLY UP,
AND BEND YUR SPINE LITTLE BACKWARDS WITH
GRACEFUL SWAYING MOTION, WHILE DOING
THE ABOVE INHALE. HOLD THE BREATH, AND
BEND FORWARD, UNTIL YOU CAN REST YOUR
ELBOWS, (THE ARMS BENT) ON THE EARTH,
THEN SWING YOUR BODY ON ELBOWS AND
KNEES UNTIL YOU CAN TOUCH THE EARTH
WITH OUR FOREHEAD. (NOTE: THE MOMENT
YOU STRIKE THE EARTH WITH YOUR ELBOWS
AND HAND RELEASE THE BREATH.)
NOW ADJUST THE FOREARMS, HANDS AND ELB-
OWS COMFORTABLY, AND STRIVE TO TOUCH
YOUR KNEES WITH THE CHIN. BREATH ACCOR
DING TO DEMANDS NATURAL WITH YOUR POS-
TURE, BUT TRY TO HOLD YOUR BREATH LONGER
DURING BREATHING, AS IT IS APT TO SEND
MORE BLOOD INTO YOUR HEAD AND FACE,
WHICH IS THE AIM OF THIS EXERCISE,
WHEN YOU FEEL ALLREADY A POWERFUL
PRESSURE WITHIN YOUR HEAD AND FACE
RISE THE UPPER PART OF THE BODY UP,
AND RISING YOUR ARMS AND HAND AS IN
THE BEGINNING OF EXERCISE SWAY SLIGH-
TLY BACKWARDS BREATHING DEEPLY. UN-
TIL YOU WILL FEEL THAT BLOOD RECEDED
FROM THE HEAD AND FACE. THEN INHALE
DEEPLY, AND BEND AGAIN, REPEATING
THE EXERCISE, AS DESCRIBED ABOVE.
DO IT FOR FIVE (5) MINUTES, BENDING,
AND STRAIGHTENING. DO IT EVERY DAY
GRADUALLY LENGHTENING THE TIME
UP TO (30) THIRTY MINUTES. NOTE: TIME
MAY VARIED ACCORDING TO NECESSITY,
AND DOING EXERCISE PAREXEMPLE FOR

FIFTEEN (15) MINUTES YOU SHOULD BEND AND
STRAIGHTEN FIFTEEN TIMES OR MORE.

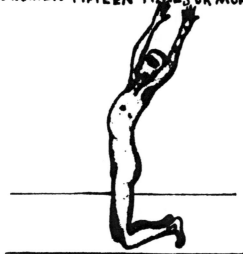

FIRST PART OF THE XII ARCANE. RAISING ON THE
KNEES AND SWAYING SLIGHTLY BACKWARDS.
SENDING BLOOD AWAY FROM HEAD AND FACE.

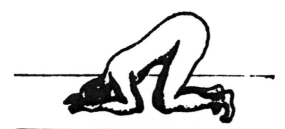

SECOND PART OF THE XII ARCANE. BENDING, PROSTRA-
TING. SENDING BLOOD TO HEAD AND FACE.

THE ABOVE IS THE REJUVENATING ARCANE
ALSO TO RENEW AND CLEAN THE TISSUES
IN DIFFERENT PARTS OF THE BODY YOU
HAVE TO LEARN THE WAY OF SENDING
THE BLOOD TO THEM, AND ALSO TO
WITHDRAW IT. IT IS DONE BY HAVING
THE CENTER OF THE PART TO BE FLUSHED
WITH BLOOD PUT BELOW THE OTHER PARTS
THEN IT WILL BE FILLED WITH BLOOD,
TO WITHDRAW THE BLOOD PUT THE CENTS
OF THE PART OF THE BODY TO BE DRAINED
OF THE BLOOD HIGHER THEN THE OTHER PARTS.
  NOTES. YOU SHOULD KNOW ALSO, THAT
WHEN INHALING THE BLOOD IS RECEEDING
FROM DIFFERENT PARTS OF THE BODY,
WHEN HOLDING THE AIR IN THE LUNGS,
AND ALSO WHEN EXHALING BLOOD
CIRCULATES STRONGER.
THE CIRCULATION, ONRUSH, AND WITHDRA-
WAL OF THE BLOOD TO AND FROM THE HEAD
IS ABSOLUTELY SYNCHRONIC WITH THE
BREATH.
THE BLOOD PRESSURE IS IN THE ARTERIES,
WHERE IS THE PURE OXYDISED BLOOD, WHICH
UNDER THIS PRESSURE REACHES THE CAPI-
LLARIES, THE CELLS, AND FEEDS THEM ALSO
GIVING THEM THE OXYGEN TO UPHOLD BURNING
OF VASTE PRODUCTS AND TRANSMUTE THEM
INTO FORM EASY TO ELIMINATE FROM THE
ORGANISM. THOSE VASTE PRODUCTS GET
INTO VENOUS BLOOD, AND ARE BURNT
OUT IN THE LUNGS, SWEATED THROUGH THE
PORES OF THE SKIN, ELIMINATED THROUGH
THE KIDNEYS, AND ALSO BOWELS AND LIVER.
IN THE VEINS BLOOD PRESSURE IS LOWER THEN
IN THE ARTERIES. THE REACH OF BLOOD TO THE
TISSUES CAN BE CONTROLLED ALSO BY

PRESSING THE ARTERIES AND VEINS.
BY PRESSING ON THE ARTERIES WE STOP THE
FLOW OF THE BLOOD TO THE PART OF THE BODY
WHERE IT IS DESTINED, AND THE BLOOD
LEFT DRAINS THROUGH THE VEINS, LEAVING
THE PART BLODLESS.
BY PRESSING ON THE VEINS, THE OUTFLOW OF
THE BLOOD IS CHECKED, BUT THE INFLOW IS
OPEN THRU THE ARTERIES, FILLING THE PART
WITH BLOOD.
 BY STUDY OF PLACES WHERE ARTERIES AND
VEINS ARE CLOSE TO THE SKIN, ONE CAN EASILY
CONTROL THE FLOW AND THE EBB OF THE BLOOD
BY PRESSING MANIPULATIONS.
ANOTHER WAY OF CONTROLLING THE CIRCULA
TION IS BY TENSING DIFFERENT SETS OF MUS-
CLES TROUGH WHICH THE VEINS AND THE
ARTERIES PASS. TENSING OF THE MUSCLES
CONTRACTS THE ARTERIES AND VEINS BY
PINCHING THEM.
 GREAT INFLVENCE ON THE HUMAN BODY
IS EXERTED BY THE FEET AND THE TOES
AND EXERCISING THE SECOND MASTER
ARCANE (GRAND) HAS VERY SERIOUS IM-
PORTANCE. (STANDING AND RISING ON
THE BALLS OF THE FEET). MASSAGE THE
FEET THOROUGLY, EXERCISWG AND KNEEDING
THE ANKLES, AND ALL THE MUSCLES OF THE
FEET, MASSAGE AND PULL THE TOES, THAN
PRESS THE TIPS OF THEM, ESPECIALLY THE
GREAT TOE, IT WILL AWAKEN NERVES, BRING
ABOUT INCREASED CIRCVLATION OF BLOOD,
AND BENEFICIALLY REACT ON THE NERVOUS
CENTERS AND GANGLIAS, STIMULATING
TROUGH THEM THE DIFFERENT GLANDS IN
THE BODY. MOVE THE ANKLES AROUND
UP AND DOWN, WITH VIGOUR, SIDEWAYS,
DO IT TOO WITH THE TOES!

BESIDES THE FEET PAY VERY STRICT ATTENTION
TO THE HANDS.
BEND YOUR ARMS IN THE ELBOWS, AND HAVE
THE HANDS BECOME ABSOLUTELY LIMP AND
RELAXED, PERFECTLY FLEXIBLE AT THE WRISTS,
SHAKE THE HANDS WITH THE MOTION OF
FOREARMS AND ARMS, UP AND DOWN, AND
THEN IN CIRCLES, WITH SO QUICK MOTION
AS TO BLURR THE VISION OF THE HANDS,
DO IT UNTIL WHEN YOU STOP YOU WILL FEEL
THE STRONG VIBRATION IN YOUR HANDS,
COMPARABLE TO THE ELECTRIC CURRENT.
RUB THE HANDS STRONGLY TOGETHER IN EVERY
WAY, THAN BEND INWARDS AND OUTWARDS
THE FINGERS AND PALMS, PRESSING THEM
TOGETHER, ALSO MOVE THUMBS AWAY FROM
THE FINGERS PRESSED TOGETHER AND TRY
TO STRETCH THE DIFFERENCE BETWEEN
THEM AND THE OTHER FINGERS BY PRESSING.

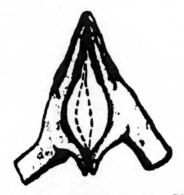

STRETCHING AND STRENGHTE-
NING THE THUMBS.

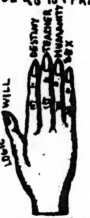

MEANING OF THE
FINGERS.

THIS EXERCISE DEVELOPES THE THUMBS,

AND DEVELOPING THEM GROWS AND STRENGH-
TENS THE WILLPOWER.
(ABOVE IS GIVEN THE CONNECTION BETWEEN
THE FINGERS AND ATTRIBUTES OF HUMAN
BEING. THUMB IS LOGIC AND WILL POWER,
INDEX FINGER IS DESTINY (COMMAND),
MIDDLE FINGER IS TEACHERS (USED
IN DRAWING ON THE SAND, AND FOR
EXPLAINING), THIRD FINGER IS HUMANI-
TARIAN LOVE, COMPASSION, AND ALTRUISM,
LITTLE FINGER IS SEX, LUST, PHYSICAL
LOVE.
YOU MUST LEARN TO CONTROL AND MASTER
THE MOTIONS AND RELATIONS BETWEEN
THEMSELVES OF ALL THE FINGERS.
DO NOT STICK OUT THE LITTLE FINGER
IT MEANS OVER SEXUALITY.
NEVER FOLD THE THUMB UNDER THE OTHER
FINGERS WHEN MAKING A FIST, IT DENO-
TES WEAK WILL, POOR HEALTH, AND PRO
PENSITY FOR LYING.
STUDY HANDS OF OTHERS, WATCHING THEM
IN POSTURES OF THE HANDS AND FINGERS
THE FINGERS WHICH ARE UNITED BY PRES-
SING TOGETHER EMPHASIS THE ATTRIBU-
TES ASCRIBED TO THEM, UNLESS THEY
ARE FOLDED AGAINST THE PALM, WHEN
THE ATTRIBUTES TO BE PAID ATTEN-
TION TO WILL BE THOSE OF THE EXTEN-
DED FINGERS.)
NOW COMES THE EXERCISE FOR ELECTRI-
FYING AND MAGNETISING OF THE HANDS
MAKING THEM POUR OUT THE HEALING
WOOFNT, USED IN PUTTING ON HANDS
TO ALLEVIATE PAIN AND STIRRING
UP THE RESTORATIVE PROCESSES IN

97

THE HUMAN BODY. —•— FACE DIR. OF SUN
STAND UP OR SIT DOWN, BACK STRAIGHT, BODY
ERECT, HEAD UP CHIN IN. EXHALE THOROU-
GHLY AND START INHALING. INHALE FOR
SEVEN SECONDS. WHILE INHALING
PUT YOUR RIGHT HAND PALM DOWN
ON YOUR LEFT HAND PALM UP AND
RUB THE PALM OF THE LEFT HAND WITH
THE PALM OF THE RIGHT, (INCLUDING
FINGERS) IN CIRCULAR MOTION FROM
RIGHT TO LEFT, MAKING DURING THE
INHALATION SEVEN CIRCLES WITH THE
RIGHT HAND, ▉▉▉ AT THE END OF
SEVENTH CIRCLE GLIDE ▉▉ YOUR RIGHT
HAND AWAY FROM YOURSELF AND YOUR
LEFT PALM WITH MOTION AS IF BRUSHING
OFF, HOLD BREATH ONE SECOND, AT THE
SAME TIME TURNING THE PALM OF
OUR LEFT HAND DOWN AND BRINGING
THE BACK OF THE HAND UP. NOW BEGN
TO EXHALE FOR SEVEN SECOND, AT THE
SAME TIME PUTTING YOUR PALM OF THE
RIGHT HAND ON THE BACK OF THE LEFT, AND
RUBBING WITH CIRCULAR MOTION FROM RIGHT
TO LEFT, MAKING DURING THE SEVEND
SECOND EXHALATION SEVEN CIRCULAR
RUBBINGS OF THE LEFT HAND.
AT THE END OF THE SEVENT MOTION GLIDE
THE RIGHT HAND AWAY FROM THE LEFT
WITH THE BRUSHING OF MOTION.
HOLD THE BREATH FOR ONE SECOND, AT THE
SAME TIME TURNING THE PALM OF YOUR
RIGHT HAND UP. NOW BEGIN TO INHALE
FOR SEVEN SECONDS, RUBBING WITH THE
PALM OF YOUR LEFT HAND, THE PALM

OF YOUR RIGHT IN CIRCULAR MOTION
OF THE LEFT HAND FROM LEFT TO RIGHT,
MAKE COMPLETE BREAT AS BEFORE
DESCRIBED, BUT USING THE RIGHT
HAND TO BE RUBBED, THEN AGAIN SWITCH
TO LEFT HAND. DO IT TWELVE TIMES
MAKING COMPLETE MASTER EXERCISE
3 MINUTES AND 12 SECOND, RUBBING EACH
HAND SIXTIMES IN VARYING SUCCESSION:
THIS COMPLETES THE MAGNETIC-ELECTRIC
EXERCISE OF THE HANDS.—

FINISHING ABOUT LAYING ON OF THE HANDS
YOU MUST KNOW THAT GIVING AND CONVE-
YING HAND IS THE RIGHT HAND, AND IT
SHOULD BE PUT ON THE SUFFERING PART
OF THE BODY, WHILE THE LEFT HAND
SHOULD BE PUT ON THE OPPOSITE SIDE FROM
PAIN, AS A RECEIVING POLE FOR THE HEA-
LING POWER.
WHEN MORE ENERGY IS NECESSARY, BEFORE
PUTTING ON OF THE HAND, DRY THEM WELL
AND HEAT BY BRISK FRICTION OF ONE AGAI
NST THE OTHER.
THE BODY CAN BE KNEEDED AND MASSAGE
VIGOUROUSLY, AS ALSO PART AFFECTED PRE
SSED STRONGLY, WHEN THERE IS NO FEVER
AND NO WOUNDS OR STRAINED TISSUES.
IN CASE OF ABOVE MENTIONED CONDITIONS
BEING PRESENT PUT HAND LIGHTLY AND
CONCENTRATE MORE ON SENDING POWER
DELICATELY, TO MEND THE BROKEN TISSUES,
AND AWAKEN THEM TO THE HEALING PROCE
WHEN EXERCISING HANDS, TO BRING HARMO-
NY INTO BODY PROCESSES, PRESS THE FINGER
TIPS OF EVERY FINGER, ███ OF ONE HAND
BETWEEN THUMB AND INDEY FINGER OF THE
OTHER HAND. PALM AND ESPECIALLY THE

MUSCLE BETWEN THE INDEX FINGER AND THE
THUMB, (UNDER THE THUMB) SHOULD BE ALSO
PRESSED.
TO CHANGE THE BLOOD PRESSURE MAKING
IT NORMAL, PUT FINGERS OF BOTH HANDS
ON THE SIDES OF THE NECK BELOW THE
BACK OF THE EARS AND MASSAGE THO-
ROUGHLY, PRESSING THEM AND MASSA-
GING WITH CIRCULAR MOTIONS.
FOR STOMACK AND SEX DISORDERS, TAKE A
WOODEN STICK 3/4" OF AN INCH WIDE AND 1/4 TO
1/2 "INCH THICK, ROUNDED ON THE END AND
THE EDGES, ABOUT 6" TO 8" INCHES LONG.

THE FORM OF THE STICK.
HAVE THE STICK WELL POLISHED. TO CURE
STOMACK CONDITIONS AND ALSO TO MAKE
BOWELS MOVE, AND IMPROVE THE GENE-
RAL TONE OF SEX ORGANS, TAKE THE
STICK AND INSERT IT INTO THE OPEN
MOUTH, LAYING IT ON THE TONGUE.
THE HOLDING IT WITH BOTH HANDS
PRESS HARD, TO MAKE THE ROUNDED
PART OF THE STICK PRESS ON THE
TONGUE. IT WILL HURT, BUT ONE HAS TO STAND
IT FROM FIVE TO FIFTEEN MINUTES.
FOR UPPER ABDOMEN PRESS AGAINST
THE ▮▮▮▮ MIDDLE OF THE TONGUE,
FOR BOWELS AND SEX, PRESS DEEP
TOWARD THE ROOT OF THE TONGUE.
CAUTION: THIS EXERCISE SHOULD NOT BE
DONE TO A PREGNANT WOMAN, AS IT
WOULD BRING ABOUT MISCARRIAGE.
THE THINGS IN ALL DESCRIBED ABOVE

100

CONSTITUTE THE ARCANE AND EXERCISES FOR
REJUVENATION OF THE HUMAN BODY, AS
WELL AS CURATIVE MEASURES, AND DEVE-
LOPEMENT FOR HEALING OF ONE ANOTHE
OTHERS, TAKING IN - BLOOD, GLANDS,
CONSCIOUS DIRECTING OF THE BLOOD
STREAM, FEET AND HANDS AND TONGUE
AND THEIR RELATIONS TO HEALTH.

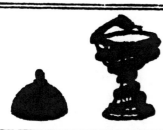

XIII L. ARCANE REJUVENATION OF ENERGY
FOR INCREASING SPAN OF
LIFE. THIS ARCANE IS TO PRACTICED
IN ▮▮▮ IMPORTANT CASES.

▮▮▮▮▮▮▮▮, BODY BATTERY OF LIFE ENERGY IS
CONCENTRATED IN THE SPINAL FLUID, AND
THE FLUID TUCHING THE CENTERS SUPPLIES
THEM WITH THE POWER OF LIFE.
HUMAN ORGANISM HAS A WAY, TO STIR UP THE
SPINAL FLUID BY NATURAL MEANS, IN CASES
OF EXHAUSTION AND LOW EBB OF ENERGIES.
THE WAY IS YAWNING. - PROCESS OF YAWNING
PRESSES ON MEDULLA OBLONGATA, AT THE
SAME TIME MAKING IT AUGMENT PRESSURE
ON THE CAVITIES IN THE HEAD, AND THE CEN-
TRAL CANAL (FOURTH VENTRICLE) IN THE SPINE,
DURING PROCESS OF SATISFACTORY YAWNING
YOU FEEL REFRESHING PRESSURE WITHIN

THE HEAD, SPREADING TOWARD THE EARS W
WHICH YOU WILL HEAR RUMBLING SOUND,
AND ALSO SOUND OF RINGING LIKE WITH DE-
LICATE SILVER CHAINS. ALSO ONE PERFORMS
A DEEP SATISFACTORY INHALATION FELT
AS PLEASANTLY FILLING ▄▄ AND PERVADING
THE SOLAR PLEXUS.

DIAGRAMS OF CAVITIES
AND ORGANS IN THE BRAIN

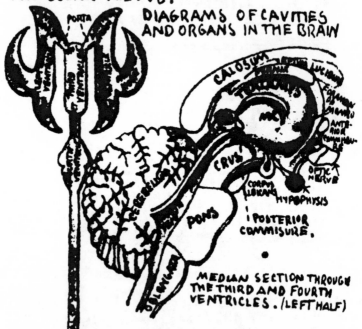

MEDIAN SECTION THROUGH
THE THIRD AND FOURTH
VENTRICLES. (LEFT HALF)

THERE ARE TWO EXERCISES BESI-
DES YAWNING WHICH CAN BE
USED FOR REDISTRIBUTING OF THE
SPINAL FLUID AND THEREBY ESTAB-
LISHING FRESH CONNECTION OF
SUPPLY OF LIFE ENERGY TO THE
NERVOUS CENTERS WITHIN THE HUMAN
BODY. THOSE TWO EXERCISES AS WELL
AS YAWNING SHOULD AND CAN BE

USED WHEN THE CIRCUMSTANCES CALL FOR
IT.

I (FIRST EXERCISE.) TENSE YOUR JAW MUSCLES
WITHOUT CLENCHING THE TEETH, (TENSING THE
MUSCLES ON THE SIDES OF THE JAW AS IF
CHEWING BUT WITHOUT CLAMPING THE TEETH
TENSE AND RELAX THE MUSCLES, SLIGHTLY
MOVING THE LOWER JAW FORWARD AND
BACKWARD. WHEN DOING IT YOU WILL HEAR
THE RING OF DELICATE SILVER CHAINS IN
YOUR EARS, THE SOUND PROVES THAT THE
EXERCISE IS DONE CORRECTLY.
REPEAT DOING IT FOR A TWELVE TIMES
OR MORE, ACCORDING TO NEED.
 THEN OPEN YOUR MOUTH AS WIDE AS
POSSIBLE, USING THE JAW MUSCLES TO
THE UTMOST. CLOSE THE EYES, PRESSING
THE EYELIDS STRONGLY TOGETHER.
YOU WILL HEAR THEN THE RUMBLING
SOUND IN YOUR EARS, AND TEARS WILL
SHOW IN YOUR EYES. THOSE ARE THE
SIGNS THAT THE EXERCISE IS DONE CORREC-
TLY. DO IT TWELVE TIMES OR MORE.
 NOW COMBINE THE FIRST PART OF
EXERCISE WITH THE SECOND, —TENSING
THE JAW MUSCLES AS IF FOR CHEWING,
AT THE SAME TIME OPENING THE
MOUTH WIDE AND CLOSING THE EYES
STRONGLY SHUT. WHILE DOING THIS
WHEN OPENING THE MOUTH, INHALE
THROUGH IT HEARTILY UNTIL YOU GET
FEELING OF SATISFACTION AND FULFIL-
MENT IN THE SOLAR PLEXUS.
DO IT TWELVE OR MORE TIMES.
IT IS RELAXING THE ENTIRE NERVOUS
SYSTEM, AND AT THE SAME TIME GIVING.

IT THE POSSIBILITY, TO BE ABLE IF NECESSA-
RY TO TENSE AGAIN ACCORDING TO THE NEW
PATTERN FOR THOUGHT.
WORK AT THIS EXERCISE, STUDY IT IN EVE-
RY WAY, AND YOU WILL DISCOVER THE ONE
MOST IMPORTANT KEY TO ENERGY AND PO-
WER.
NOTE;-YAWNING SENDS OUT TREMENDOU-
SLY POWERFUL VAWES ON THE EATHER,
INFLUENBING THE IDENTICAL ORGANS
OF PEOPLE IN PROXIMITY ▬▬ TELEPA-
THICALLY, AND MAKING THEM YAWN
IN TURN.' THAT WHY THE YAWNING IS
SO CATCHING.
BY STUDYING THIS PROCESS YOU WILL
KNOW THAT THE BEST WAY OF SENDING
OUT OF TELEPATIC MESSAGES IS TO
▬▬▬▬ BEGIN WITH YAWNING EXER-
CISE, AND AFTER COMPLETELY RELA-
XING, SENDING OUT MESSAGE VIBRA-
TIONS ON THE YAWNING BREATH.
II (SECOND EXERCISE) PUT YOUR HANDS
TOGETHER PALMS UP, FINGERS BENT SO THAT
BACKS OF THEM TUUCH, THE TIPS OF THUMBS
PRESSED AGAINST EACH OTHER⁰.

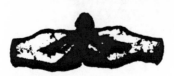

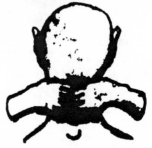

POSTURES FOF THE
SECOND EXERCISE.

NOW WITHOUT SEPARATING THE FINGERS MOVE
YOUR HAND OVER YOUR HEAD AND BACKWARD,
SO THAT THE ENDS OF YOUR BENT FINGERS WILL
REST ON THE SPOT WHERE THE HEAD JOINS
THE NECK. PRESS LIGHTLY WITH FINGERS
AGAINST THE SPOT BETWEEN THE HEAD
AND THE NECK. MOVE THE HEAD DOWN
WARDS RESTING YOUR CHIN ON YOUR
CHEST, THEN LIFTED AND MOVE IT UP-
WARDS AND BACKWARDS, WITHOUT
REMOVING THE PRESSURE OF FINGERS
AND HANDS. AGAIN REPEAT THE MO-
VEMENT OF THE HEAD TO REST THE
CHIN ON THE CHEST, AND CONTINUE DO-
ING IT TWELVE TIMES OR MORE.
THIS EXERCISE HAS A GREAT INFLUENCE
ON MEDULLA OBLONGATA OR PINEAL
GLAND DEVELOPING ITS SIZE AND CAPACITY.
THIS EXERCISE CAN AND SHOULD BE DONE
FOR THE DEVELOPEMENT ACCORDING TO THE
NEED FOR THE EXPANSION OF ENERGIES.
NOTE: DURING THE EXERCISE YOU CAN STAND OR
SIT, WITH THE SPINE ERECT. AS TO THE PO-
SITION OF THE FINGERS ON THE POINT BET-
WEEN HEAD AND NECK, THE MIDDLE FINGER
SHOULD BE RIGHT ON THE SPOT, OTHERS ACCOR-
DINGLY ON THE SIDES.
DURING THIS EXERCISE OR IMMEDIATELY AFTER
YOU CAN FEEL AND HEAR THE HISSING SOUND
OF VIBRATION AT THE BASE OF THE SKULL. -
THIS IS RESULT OF PERCOLATING OF THE SPINAL
FLUID, TO AND FROM THE FOURTH VENTRI-
CLE.
NOW COMES THE EXERCISE, WHICH HAS A
TREMEDOUS IMPORT IN THE DEVELOPEMENT,
AND WHICH IS HARD TO EXPLAIN, WITHOUT
PRACTISING AND UNDERSTANDING THE

ABOVE DESCRIBED EXERCISES. IT IS THE
PRINCIPLE WHICH ENTITLES ONE TO BE ONE OF
THE ORDER OF THE ~~SERPENT~~.
SIT DOWN OR STAND UP, SPINE STRAIGHT, BODY
ERECT HEAD UP CHIN IN.
TAKE INHALATION, AND LOCK THE PASSAGE OF THE
AIR IN THE THROAT, (USING LARYNX), THEN TENSE
INSIDE OF YOU, (DIAPHRAGM), AS IF YOU WOULD
WANT TO HAVE A STOOL. NOW RISE THE
TENSION FROM THE LOWER BOWEL UP,
—RELAXING LOWER BOWEL, TENSING
STOMACH; RELAXING STOMACH, TENSING
AROUND INSIDE OF THE THROAT,—
CONCENTRATE ON THE FEELING OF PRES-
SURE IN THE BACK OF THE HEAD. IN FACT
CONCENTRATE ON THIS FEELING FROM
THE BEGINNING OF THE EXERCISE.
THE MOMENT YOU NEED THE AIR EXHALE AND
INHAL FREELY AND EASILY, YOU WILL NOTICE
THAT THE TENSION IN YOUR HEAD BEGINNING
AT THE BASE OF THE SKULL CAN BE KEPT
EVEN WHEN YOU ARE BREATHING. STUDY
THIS PROCESS, SO THAT YOU CAN TENSE
YOUR MEDULLA AT WILL, AND ALSO RE-
LAX IT BY WILL. NOTICE THAT DURING THE
TENSING, MUSCLE BEETWEEN THE BASE
OF THE SKULL AND THE NECK TENSES
ALSO, PUT YOUR FINGER TIPS ON IT AND
STUDY THE DIFFERENT DEGREES OF
TENSION IN THIS MUSCLE ON THE BACK OF
YOUR NECK, YOU WILL FIND OUT THAT
YOU CAN RELAX THIS MUSCLE AND STILL
FEEL THE PRESSURE IN THE HEAD.
WHEN YOU ARE RELAXING THE TENSENESS IN
YOUR HEAD, MOVE YOUR HEAD BACKWARDS
AND FORWARDS, SIDEWAYS TO THE RIGHT

AND TO THE LEFT, SHAKE THE FACE TO RIGHT
AND TO LEFT, AND SIMPLY ROLL YOUR HEAD
ON YOUR SHOULDERS, - THOSE ARE MOTIONS
THAT WILL HELP TO RELAX THE TENTION IN
THE MEDULLA OBLONGATA AND THE HEAD.
USE THIS EXERCISE OFTEN AND STUDY THE
FEELING CONNECTED WITH TENSION
AND RELAXATION IN THE HEAD.
FIND OUT THAT YOU CAN TENSE AT THE
BASE OF THE SKULL, (THE BACK OF THE HEAD)
THEN IN THE FRONT OF THE HEAD - BACK OF
THE POINT BETWEEN THE EYEBROWS, THEN
ON THE TOP OF THE HEAD, - ALSO YOU WILL
FIND THAT YOU CAN IN YOUR CONSCIOUSNESS
SEPARATE THOSE AREAS AND KEEP THEM
TENSE - ONE AT THE TIME. PRACTICE THE
TENSING OF THE RIGHT SIDE AND THE LEFT
WITHIN YOUR HEAD. DO THIS PRACTICE
DILIGENTLY, SLOWLY AND PERSISTENTLY.
KEEP YOUR CONSCIOUSNESS AT ALL THE
TIMES ALERT FOR THE PHENOMENA
GOING ON INSIDE YOUR HEAD AND THE -
BRAIN.
NOTE. THE TENSENESS IS RECOGNIZED
BY FEELING OF PRESSURE WITHIN.
ALWAYS AFTER EXERCISING RELAX IN-
SIDE OF YOUR HEAD COMPLETELY, BY
MOVING YOUR HEAD ON THE NECK.

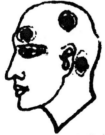

AREAS OF TENSION
PRESSURE FELT INSIDE
OF THE HEAD.
LEARN TO KNOW THOSE
POINTS WITHIN YOURSELF
THE ARE THE KEYS AND
THE LOCKS TO KNOWLEDGE
OF YOURSELF.

THIS EXERCISE DEVELOPES THE PINEAL GLAND

(MEDULLA OBLONGATA) AND GIVES YOU STRAIGHT
PATH IN SELFREALISATION AND MASTERY.
IT HAS TO BE EXPLAINED HERE THAT THE
THOUGHT IS FORMED (ELECTRICALLY) IN
MAGNETICALLY TENSED FORMATION IN
THE BRAIN, WHICH MAGNETICAL TEN-
SION CAN BE RELAXED OF TENSED THRU
THE WORK OF MEDULLA OBLONGATA.
THE SOUL AS A ETERNAL I, I AM, -
WITH THE ATTRIBUTES - I THINK, I FEEL
I WILL IS REVOLVING BETWEEN THE
THREE POINTS IN THE HEAD, BEING
ALWAYS IN THE PRESENT, BUT TRAN-
SMUTING THE FUTURE INTO THE PAST.
TIME FOR THE SOUL IS NONEXISTENT.
CAUTION, IF DURING THE EXER-
CISE YOU FIND THAT YOUR HEAD
BEGINS TO VIBRATE SIDEWAYS, -
(SHAKING MOTION) IT MEANS THAT
THE ENERGY IS PENT UP TO THE POINT OF
OVERFLOWING, AND IS GETTING OF ON THE
ETHER, THEN YOU MUST STOP THE EXER-
CISE AND RELAX.
THE ABOVE COMPRISES THE EXER-
CISES WHICH CAN AND SHOULD BE DONE,
TO DEVELOPE CENTERS IN THE HEAD, ES-
PECIALLY THE MEDULLA OBLONGATA OR
SOCALLED OTHERWISE PINEAL GLAND.
IT IS CONSTITUTING THE L. ARCANE XIII.
, IN VERY IMPORTANT AND RARE
CASES, WHEN LIFE IS AT STAKE, AND THE
ENERGY WITHIN THE SPINAL FLUID IS LOW,
ON ACCOUNT OF DEFICIENCY OF YOUTH-
FULLNESS IN THE SAME AND ALSO NOT
SUFFICIENT AMOUNT OF IT, A OPERATION
CAN BE PERFORMED FOR REPLENISHING.

THE LACK AND QUALITY, OF SPINAL FLUID.
YOU MUST HAVE FOR THIS THE ASSISTANCE OF
A TRUSTWORTHY INITIATED PUPIL OR DASMTR
A YOUNG, HEALTY PERSON OF THE SAME BLOOD
LIKE YOU SHOULD BE CHOSEN, AND BE LOVINGLY
WILLING TO HELP YOU WITH ITS OWN LIVING
SPINAL FLUID. THE PUNCTURE WITH A SYRINGE
EQUIPPED WITH A HOLLOW NEEDLE SHOULD BE
DONE, DRAWING THE SPINAL FLUID FROM
BETWEEN THE VERTEBRAS OF THE SPINAL
COLUMN. AMOUNT TAKEN FROM YOU SHOLD
BE LITTLE, ONLY TO ESTABLISH THE CONTACT
BETWEEN YOUR SPINAL CANAL. AMOUNT
TAKEN FROM OTHER PERSON SHOULD BE
BIGGER ACCORDING TO THE NEEDS AND
THE NECESSITY, PAYING STRICTEST ATTE-
NTION NOT TO INJURE ▬ IN ANY WAY
THE DONOR.— BOTH SPINAL FLUIDS —YOURS AND
DONORS ARE MIXED TOGETHER AND INJECTED
IN YOU NEAR THE PUNCTURE IN YOUR SPINE.

XIV L. ARCANE. DEMAND, COMMAND.

STRIVING TO ATTAIN THE THINGS IN LIFE, REALISE
YOUR CORRELATION TO IT.- SIT DOWN AT THE DESK
OR TABLE FACING IN THE DIRECTION OF THE SUN.
RELAX, AND CONCENTRATE ON THE SELF-RE-
ALISATION.- I - I AM.- PONDER ON THE TRUTH
OF YOUR BEING, CONSIDER THE ATTRIBUTES
OF YOUR EGO - I THINK, I FEEL, I-WILL.
FEEL YOURSELF BEING CONSCIOUS OF YOUR-
SELF, WITHIN THE CENTER OF YOUR BRAIN
RECEIVING THE IMPRESSIONS AND TRAN-
SMITING THEM INTO THE EXPRESSIONS,
HAVE A CLEAR CONCEPTION AND UNDERSTANDING OF
THE WORDS- „I CAN „„I WANT „„I MUST„„I WILL„
CONCENTRATE ON THE OBJECT OF YOUR DESIRE.
IMAGINE IT CLEARLY AND PLAINLY,- FEEL YOUR
DESIRE IN YOUR SOLAR PLEXUS.-
WHEN THE REALISATION OF THE INEVITABLE
NESS OF YOUR DESIRE WILL DAWN UPON
YOU- INWOKE THE PASSWORD WHICH IS
DETERMINATION.
INHALE DEEPLY AND HOLD YOUR BREATH
LOCKING IT WITH PHARYNX. LIFT YOUR RIGH
HAND CLOSING THE FIST. (THE THUMB CO-
VERING THE OTHER FINGERS), TENSE THE
FIST AND THE ARM.
NOW SUDDENLY AND WITH POWER BRI-
NG THE ARM AND THE CLOSED TENSE FIST
DOWN ON THE DESK OR TABLE, AT THE
MOMENT OF STRIKING RELAXING THE
FIST AND RELEASING THE AIR FROM THE
LUNGS. USE WITH EXHALATION THE
WORDS-„I DEMAND„ OR „I COMMAND„
STATING THE WISH.- WHEN THE
FIST IS BROUGHT DOWN, LET IT BOU-
NCE FROM THE DESK OR THE TABLE
IN SEMICIRCULAR MOTION TOWARD

YOURSELF, AND FINISH WITH SHORT SHARP
SEMICIRCLE ALSO TOWARD YOURSELF.
YOU STRIKE WITH SIDE OF THE FIST OF THE
LITTLE FINGER.
REPEAT THIS EXERCISE FOR SOMETIME
ACCORDING TO THE IMPORTANCE OF YOUR
WISH.
POUNDING ON THE FLAT SURFACE DESK, TABLE
ETC.) WITH THE FIST, TOGETHER WITH WITHHOL-
DING OF THE BREATH UNTIL THE STROKE IS
POUND, SHAKES THE SOLAR PLEXUS, TRAN-
SMUTING THE IMAGE OF THE DESIRE INTO
THE HEAD, WHERE IT IS WILLIFIED, AND
IN THE FORM OF POWERFUL INVOCA-
TION (COMMAND), SENDT OUT AS RIPPLES
ON THE ETHER.
NOTE: WHEN POUNDING BEND SLIGHTLY
FOFWAR JUMPING SLIGHTLY IN RESPONSE
TO STRIKING, IN YOUR SOLAR PLEXUS,
HAUNCHES AND HEAD.
THIS ENDS THE XIV ARCANE, FOR DEMAND
AND COMMAND.
IT IS NOT NECESSARY OF EVER USING THIS AR-
CANE IN FRONT OF OTHERS. YOU SHOULD DO
IT ALONE.
BUT WHEN NECESSITY ARISES TO USE IT ON
HUMAN BEING DIRECTLY, DO IT IN A DI-
FFERENT FORM. REMEMBERING THE
INSIDE WORK OF THIS ARCANE, DO IT ONLY
MENTALLY, AS A SUBSTITUTE FOR POUNDING
USING UNNOTICEABLE PRESSURE FOR EM-
PHASIS, THERE ARE THREE WAYS OF DOING IT.
FIRST HOLD WITH YOUR RIGHT HAND, THE WRIST
OF THE LEFT. UPPER PART OF THE RIGHT HAND
EXPOSED, THE PALM COVERING THE UPPER
PART OF LEFT HAND, AND FINGERS OF THE
RIGHT HAND GRASPING THE LEFT WRIST.

111

SECOND: INSTEAD OF CLASPING THE LEFT WRIST
CLASP THE OUTER SIDE OF LEFT HAND, SO THAT
THE THUMB OF THE RIGHT HAND WILL PRESS
ON THE LEFT WRIST, (OUTSIDE), AND THE REST
OF THE FINGERS OF THE RIGHT HAND WILL
PRESS IN THE HOLLOW OF THE LEFT PALM.
THIRD: BEND THE FINGERS OF THE RIGHT AND
LEFT HANDS TOGETHER AND HOOK THE BOTH
HANDS SO THAT THE BENT FINGERS OF THE
RIGHT AND LEFT HAND WILL PRESS AND
TOUCH ON THEIR INSIDE, WHILE THE THUMBS WILL
BE ON THE OUTSIDE TOUCHING THE KNUCKLES OF
THE FINGERS FROM THE OUTSIDE.

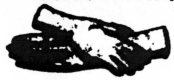

FIRST POSITION

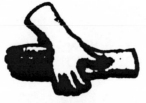

SECOND POSITION

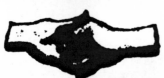

THIRD POSITION

THE COMMAND OR DEMAND SHOULD BE SPOKEN
IN A QUIET VOICE, CHARGING IT WITH POWER,
AND PUTTING STRESS ON WORDS EXACTLY CON.
VEYING THE WISH. DURING COMMANDING BENT.
HAND SHOULD BE IMPERCEPTIBLY TIGHTENED
UPON THE LEFT, IN THE THIRD POSITION
REMEMBER MEANING OF THE FINGERS

I.E. TUMB - THE WILL ; INDEX-DESTINY-COM-MAND ; MIDDLE FINGER-TEACHER-CONWE YOR ; FOURTH FINGER-HUMANE FEELINGS - SYMPATHY-ALTRUISM ; LITTLE FINGER-SEX -CARNAL DESIRE. ACCORDING TO FEELINGS YOU WANT TO AWAKE AND COMMAND, PRESS -WITH THE THUMBS ON KNUBLES OF THE FINGERS HAVING DESIRED ATTRIBUTES.

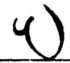

YPL. ARCANE. ESTABLISHING A MENTAL CONNE CTION WITH THE PERSON PRESENT OR ABSENT AT ANY GIVEN TIME THE BREATH , IN ITS DEPT AND ITS RHYTM SHOWS THE VIBRATION IN WHICH THE PERSON IS AT A GIVEN TIME . WHEN YOU WANT TO TUNE IN ON THE VI-BRATION OF THE PERSON FOR MAKING A INNER CONTACT, WATCH FALLING AND RISING OF THE CHEST OF THE PERSON YOU ARE CONTAC-TING , AND ACCORDINGLY START BREATHING IN UNISON. THIS WILL PUT YOU IN CONTACT WITH THE PERSON , AND YOU CAN THEN UNDERSTAND AND INFLUENCE ACCORDING TO YOUR WILL . YOU WILL FIND THAT ONCE TUNED IN YOU · CAN BY CONSCIOUS MODIFICATION OF YOUR BRE. ATH , CHANGE THE BREATH OF THE OTHER PERSON IN THIS WAY CREATING THE STATES DESIRED . DO IT WITHOUT HAVING OTHERS NOTICE THE EXERCISE . REMEMBER THAT THE HIGHEST RHYTM IS MASTER RHYTM - INHALATION SEVEN SECONDS , PAUSE ONE SECOND , EXHALATION SEVEN SECONDS PAUSE ONE SECOND. BY THIS BREATH YOU TUNE YOURSELF AND OTHERS ON THE MASTER

■ THOUGHT, AND RHYTM OF THE GEOIC ENTITY.
HAVING MANY PEOPLE AROUND IF YOU WANT
MAKE THE VIBRATE TOGETHER TUNE THEM
BY IN UNISON SINGING OF „AUM„ -
FOR A PERIOD OF FIVE TO FIFTEEN MINUTES
YOU CAN TUNE THEM ON MASTER RHYTM
BY HAVING THEM SING - YAT-HA-AH-
HU-VAI-RI-O , WHEN EXHALING,
AND INHALE FOR SEVEN SECONDS.
USE YOUR SINGING MANTRAS ACCORDING
TO THE RESULTS YOU WANT TO CREATE.
SLOWING THE VIBRATIONS CALMS, RE-
LAXES, BRINGS IN SERENITY - IT IS DONE
BY USING LONG SONOROUS MANTRAMS.
QUICKENING THE VIBRATIONS TENSES, HARDENS
THE BRAIN, BRINGS IN HYSTERICAL STATE
OFTEN ENDING IN FANATICAL UPHEAVALS,
IT INFLUENCES PSYCHIC AND SEX.
 MOST OF THE PEOPLE ARE MORE PRONE
TO QUICKER VIBRATIONS , AND IT IS MUCH
EASIER TO ACHIEVE. EXHAUSTION FOLLO-
WING THOSE STATES ONLY THEN BRINGS
RELAXATION AS A REACTION.
IN SLOW VIBRATION SWAYING MAY BE USED,
IN FAST VIBRATION CLAPPING OF HAND AND
STAMPING OF FEET.
 USE SIMPLE TUNES, AND RHYTMS.
NOTE: THE PEOPLE THAT LOVE EACH-OTHER,
TUNE IN ON EACH OTHER VIBRATION BY KISSING
CORRECT KISS IS DONE HOLDING THE BREATH
SO THAT, AFTER PERFORMING IT THEY
START BREATHING IN UNISON. ■■■■■
HELP IN TUNING IN IS HOLDING HANDS.
ESTABLISHING A MENTAL CONNECTION
AT A DISTANCE YOU MUST PICK OUT THE
TIME WHEN THE PERSON WITH WHICH YOU
WANT TO CONNECT IS IN THE RELAXED

STATE. IT IS THE BEST IN THE NIGHT TIME WHEN THE PERSON IS ASLEEP. YOU TUNE IN BY CONSCIOUSLY PUTTING YOURSELF IN RELAXED CONDITION, AND BREATHING QUIETLY AS IF ASLEEP, MENTALLY CONCENTRATING ON THE PERSON. (FOR ESTABLISHING BETTER CONTACT YOU CAN USE, SOMETHING BELONGING TO THE PERSON AND HAVING THE IMPRINT OF PERSON VIBRATIONS. (RECORD LEFT BY THE EMANATIONS OF THE ENTITY ON THE OBJECTS) ALSO A FIGURE REPRESENTING PERSON CAN BE MADE - BEING DONE WITH CONSTANT THOUGH AND FEELING OF IT BEING TRUE REPRESENTATION OF THE PERSON, AND AFTER BEING FINISHED ADORNED WITH THINGS BELONGING TO THE PERSON.

HOLDING THINGS OF THIS TYPE YOU ESTABLISH CONNECTION QUICKLY BY FOLLOWING THE THREAD - (INVISIBLE TIE) THAT BINDS THE PERSON TO THE OBJECT. TREAT THE OBJECT AS THE PERSON, WHICH GETS TO BE SO.

WHEN YOU WILL TUNE IN YOU WILL KNOW FOR THE REPRESENTATION OF THE PERSON WILL SPARKLE WITH THE LIFE OF ITS OWN, - WILL BECOME THIS PERSON.

TUNE IN DELICATLY MODULATING THE RHYTM OF YOUR BREATH, AND AFTER TUNING IN, TAKE LEAD IN ESTABLISHING YOUR TREND OF RHYTM DESIRED. (FACE DIRECTION OF THE SUN)

DO IT ONLY ACCORDING TO THE HIGHEST SPIRIT, CONSCIOUS, AND UNDERSTANDING THAT YOU ARE ACTING IN ACCORDANCE WITH THE HIGHEST WILL. THIS EXERCISE IS NOT TO BE PLAYED WITH, AND NOT FOR CURIOSITY SAKE, DO IT TO HELP.

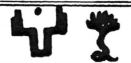

XVI LARCANE. BIRTH CONTROL AND CONTROL OF
THE SEX OF THE CHILD TO BE BORN. CONCEPTION
AND PREDESTINATION.
INTERCOURSE BETWEEN THE TWO SEXES IS THE
CREATIVE ACT OF UTMOST IMPORTANCE IT IS THE
CREATION, AND ACCORDING TO THE LAWS OF NA-
TURE IT IS KEY TO IMMORTALITY AND A ELEMENT
LINK IN THE EQUATION STARTED BY THE ANCIENT
ONES. SOUND CONVEYS THE SPARK WITH WHICH
THE SOUL TO BE INCARNATED BLEMOS AND IS ABLE
TO ESTABLISH ITSELF IN THE FLESH.
WHEN THE MAN IS SPENNING HE WILL EMIT A
SOUND MOST OF THE TIMES DOUBLE, FIRST DEEP IN-
TAKE OF THE BREATH WITH A GASP OR HISSING,
HOLDING THE BREATH AT THE MOMENT OF SPEN-
DING, AND AT THE END OF IT, EXHALING WITH
A SIGH OR A MOAN. FINAL SOUND OF EXHA-
LATION IS ?:. "OM" - CONVEYS THE SPARK
OF LIFE FROM MAN INTO THE WOMAN, PRE-
PARING THE ACT OF CONCEIVING, FERTILISATION
OF THE OVUM BY SPERMATOSOA. - WITHOUT
THIS SOUND THE CONCEIVING WON'T TAKE PLACE.
THE PREDESTINATION OF THE SEX OF CHILD TO
BE CONCEIVED DEPENDS ON THE STATE IN WHICH
PARENTS ARE AT THE TIME OF COPULATION.
IF BEFORE THE INTERCOURSE THE MAN AND WO-
MAN WILL PET AND CARESS EACH OTHER LAYING
ALONGSIDE, THE SEX OF CHILD FROM THIS UNION
WILL DEPEND ON THE BREATH IN WHICH THEY
ARE AT THE TIME OF COPULATION. - SUN OR
MOON.
WHEN THE MAN IS LAYING ON HIS LEFT SIDE
FACING THE WOMAN WHO IS LAYING ON HER
RIGH SIDE HE WILL BE IN THE SUN BREATH,
BREATH FLOWING STRONGER IN HIS RIGHT
NOSTRIL, AS HE WILL BE IN THE MOON
BREATH, BREATH FLOWING IN HER LEFT
NOSTRIL. - CHILD OF THIS UNION WILL BE
MALE.
WHE THE MAN IS LAYING ON HIS RIGHT
SIDE FACING THE WOMAN LAYING ON HER

LEFT SIDE, HE WILL BE IN THE MOON BREATH,
BREATH FLOWING IN HIS LEFT NOSTRIL, AND
THE WOMAN WILL BE IN THE SUN BREATH,
FLOWING THRU HER RIGHT NOSTRIL. —
— CHILD OF THIS UNION WILL BE FEMALE,
ACCORDING TO OTHER COMBINATIONS THAT
MAY BE CREATED — IF MAN IS IN SUN BREATH
AND SO IS THE WOMAN, OR REVERSE — THE
MALE CHILD WILL BE EFFEMINATE, OR
FEMALE CHILD WILL BE MASCULINE.
THIS ABOVE ENDS THE XVI ARCANE OF
CONTROL AND PREDESTINATION OF THE
SEX OF THE OFFSPRING FROM THE SEXUAL
UNION OF MAN AND WOMAN.

ILLUMINATION. (CONCLUSION)

YOU ARE THE MATHEMATICAL AND GEO-
METRICAL CENTER OF ALL THE UNIVERSE,
WHERE THE CENTRE IS YOU, AND RADIUS
GOES INTO THE INFINITY. INSTEAD OF GO-
ING AFTER THINGS COMMAND THEM
TO COME TO YOU. YOU ARE THE LORD IN
YOUR UNIVERSE WHICH IS _THE_ UNIVERSE,
DESIRE, WISH AND WILL, ORDER, DEMAND
COMMAND.
THIS IS THE RIDDLE OF GOD — BEING, EXISTING
EVERYPLACE, EVERYWHERE AT THE SAME
TIME.
THE MOMENT YOU REALISE AND BECOME
FULLY CONSCIOUS THAT YOU ARE THE CENTRE
OF THE UNIVERSE, YOU ARE THAT CENTRE.

CENTRE OF CENTRES MANIFESTS IN YOU, OR
YOU MANIFEST IN IT. YOU ARE ENDOWED
WITH THE GREATEST POWERS AND YOUR
POTENTIALITIES ARE INFINITE.
YOU ARE CONNECTED WITH EVERYTHING
TROUGH THE FINEST MESH OF ATTRA-
CTIONS AND REPULSIONS, AND ARE LIKE
SPIDER IN THE CENTRE OF THE WEBB
FELING AND RECEIVING THE IMPRESSIONS
FROM EVERYTHING EVERYWHERE AND
ADJUSTING THE EQUILIBRIUM OF FORCES,
 WORK, BE CONSCIOUS, DEVELOP AND
STRENGHTEN THE REALISATION —
— " I AM THE CENTRE OF THE UNI-
VERSE " — THIS IS ONENESS THIS IS
REALISATION.
 AUTHORITY, POWER, CONFIDENCE, SPRING
OUT OF THIS KNOWLEDGE, — THE REALISA-
TION OF WHICH IS THE TRUTH.
 WISDOM IS KNOWING THE TRUTH CON-
SCIUSLY.
 ALWAYS BE CONSCIOUS OF THE FACT
THAT YOU ARE THE CENTRE OF THE
UNIVERSE. " I, I AM " IS THE MAJEST
OF DIGNITY, THE ANSWER TO THE RIDDL
OF THE SIMPLICITY IN COMPLEXITIES,
 SELF REALISATION. ANSWER TO THE
GREAT DOGMA — " KNOW THYSELF ".
ANSWER TO ENIGMA — " GOD IS IMMOR-
TAL MAN — MAN IS MORTAL GOD ".
 YOU DO NOT MOVE, WHEN YOU WALK OR
RIDE, THE SOROUNDINGS MOVE ACCORDING
TO THE LAWS OF THE EQUILIBRIUM,
ADJUSTING THEMSELVES IN PROPOR-
TIONS OF ETERNAL POSITIVES AND

NEGATIVES, THE NAME FOR WHICH IS MO-
TION. YOU BECOME MANIFEST IN PLA-
CES, FACING TASKS OF ADJUSTMENT, THRU
TRANSMUTATION OF IMPRESSION INTO THE
EXPRESSION.
THIS IS MAGICK, THIS IS THE MIRACLE.
I AM THAT I AM.
AWAKEN, OPEN YOUR EYES, ARISE, BECOME
CONSCIOUS — REALISE-"I",,"I AM""I AM I"
INTERPOSING, MEASURING THE COSMIC
CONSCIOUSNES WITH SELFCONSCIUSNESS.
THE MICROCOSMOS PUTTING ON THE ROBE OF
THE MACROCOSMOS, THE MYSTERY OF THE
GREAT IN THE SMALL AND THE SMALL IN THE
GREAT.
"MY NAME IS I, MY NAME IS MANY, I AM ALL AND
I AM PART OF ALL".
WHEN FEELING OF "I" GROWS IN ONE IT IS
SELFCENTERING, - GROWTH AND DEVELOP-
MENT OF EGO. AT CERTAIN POINT OCC-
URS SATURATION FOR GIVEN PERSONALITY
BUT ACCORDING TO THE LAW - THE LIKE'
ATTRACTS ALIKE, THE GROWTH OF "I"
ONCE STARTED WILL AUGMENT TO UNEN-
DERSTENDABLE SIZE. AFTER REACHING
THE SATURATION POINT WITHIN THE BODY,
OVERFLOW OF EGO BEGINS TO EXTERNA-
LISE, OCCUPYING IN A VIBRATORY WAY
THE PLACE MUCH LARGER THEN THE BODY-
- IT REACHES OUT DISTENDING AURA, AND
CREATES WHAT THE INITIATES BEHOLD
AND UNINITIATES FEEL AS PERSONA-
LITY. EGO OF THIS DYNAMIC TYPE MER-
GES OTHER SMALLER EGOS WITHIN ITS

SCOPE OF ATTRACTION AND THIS WAY EXPANDS
STILL FARTHER. THIS IS THE EGO OF LEA-
DERS AND EXECUTIVES, AND VOLITIONARY
VIBRATION OF ITS POWER IS FELT BY THE
MULTITUDES, TUNED TO IT BY FORCE OR
BY SYMPATHY.
ORIGINALLY THE "I" THE EGO IS SMALL
WITHIN THE BODY, A IOTA, A SPARK, WHICH
IS DWELLING WITHIN, GETTING STRONGER
TROUGH THE EXERCISES OF RECEIVING
THE IMPRESSIONS AND WRESTLING WITH
THEM TO TRANSMUTE THEM INTO THE
EXPRESSIONS, PURIFYING THE CHANNELS
THAT CONWEY THE FLOOD OF MESSAGES,
AND OPENING THE WAYS THAT ANSWERS
THEM WITH A MESSAGE "I AM HERE
I AM THE PART OF ALL, I TAKE MY SHA-
KE IN THE CREATION".
UNTIL THE CHANNELS ARE ABSOLUTELY
OPEN AND PURE THIS SPARK OF I RE-
MAINS WITHIN, AND THE BODY, EXTER-
NAL PART OF IT IS THE OUTSIDE, WHILE
THE OUTSIDE FROM THE BODY IS FAR
AWAY. - THIS IS THE FIRST STAGE IN THE
DEVELOPMENT OF EGO.
SECOND STAGE IS SATURATION, TROUGH
EXERCISING AND DEVELOPMENT EGO THE
I, GROWS AND REACHES THE BOUND PRE-
SCRIBED BY THE LIMITS OF THE FLESH,
THE EGO IS AT ONE WITH THE BODY,
A PERFECT FIT, IT IS UNITY, THE SEED
GROWN TO THE SIZE OF ITS CONTAINER,

THE EGO FILLING THE VESSEL — " EAT OF THE
BREAD IT IS FLESH OF MINE, DRINK OF THE
VINE IT IS BLOOD OF MINE. "
A STAGE OF THE SAINT.
EXPANSION OF THE I, THE EGO OVERLAPS THE
BOUNDS OF THE FLESH, EGO BECOMES THE
OUTSIDE, WHILE THE BODY BECOMES THE SEED
ON THE INSIDE, THIS IS IMMORTALITY,
THE WAY OF THE GODS. EGO GRASPS
THINGS UNHEARD OF AND UNIMAGINED
BY THE UNINITIATED. — IT IS THE STAGE
OF MASTERS AND SAVIOURS, — BENT ON
SOLVING THE KARMA OF NATIONS AND
RACES ON THIS EARTH.
SUCH AN EGO THINKS, FEELS AND ACTS
TROUGH THE OTHER EGOS, THAT ARE
INCORPORATED WITHIN ITS SCOPE OF
INFLUENCE. — IT IS THE MASTER OVER THEM,
CONSCIOUS EVER WATCHFUL RECEIVING -
TRANSMUTING AND EXPRESSING TROUGH
ITS WISDOM OF CAREFUL OBSERVATION
CORRECT INTERPRETATION AND PRACTICAL
APPLICATION.
IT THINKS ON THE OUTSIDE AND SO IT
FEELS AND ACTS.. BEING CONNECTED WITH
THE OTHERS TROUGH THE INVISIBLE THREADS
OF " THE TIE THAT BINDS " IT THINKS ██
THEN ████████████ IN (ABSTRACT) SPACE,
FEELING THE THINKING NOT WITHIN
THE HEAD BUT ABOVE AT 30° OR 45°
DEGREES. PROCESS OF THINKING
FEELING, WILLING IS DONE IN

SPACE, WITH PHYSICAL BODY SERVING
ONLY AS A ROOT, A EMBRYO—" I AM
THE VINE, YE ARE THE BRANCHES."
   PROCESSES OF THOUGHT, FEELING
AND WILL GO ON FAR AHEAD OF THE
BODY, WITH FULL CONSCIOUSNESS
AND AUTORITY FOR THE ONE "/ SCA-
TTERED AROUND BUT UNITED BY THE INVI-
SIBLE TIES OF THE IDEAL RECOGNSED
BY THE OVERSOUL — THIS IS THE WAY OF AR-
HATS. " I AND MY FATHER ARE ONE."
   DEVELOPMENT OF CONSCIOUSNESS AND
EGO, MEETING ▇ HUMAN BEINGS RE-
COGNISES THE STAGES OF THEIR DE-
VELOPMENT AND CALLS THEM :-
   NEIGHBORS, FRIENDS AND FAITH-
FUL FRIENDS ACCORDING TO THEIR
INNER TRUE SELF, WHICH CAN NOT BE
HIDD FROM THE ALL SEEING EYE
FAITFUL FRIENDS BURN THE WILL LIGHT. TO SHOW THE WAY.

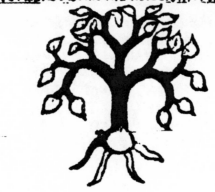

122

MAGICAL PROJECTION

INVOCATION OF THE HOST OF ANGELS OR POWERS.

CONFIRM THE " I " AND " I AM ", STAND IN A CIRCLE WITH A SQUARE INSIDE OR OUT-SIDE. SQUARE AND THE CIRCLE ARE OPE-NING THE WAY ON THE INFINITY.

FACE THE NORTH AT MIDNIGHT (CHARGE YOUR BODY WITH POWERS ACCORDING TO THE I ST MASTER ARCANE BEFORE STAR-TING THE PROJECTION).

HAVE A ALTAR IN FRONT OF YOU WITH SAME DESIGN AS THE MAGICAL CIRCLE.

ALTAR SHOULD BE BUILT FROM MARBLE, WOOD, OR METALS. DESIGNS ON IT SHOULD BE ENGRAVED, ETCHED, PAINTED OR DRAWN THE MAGICAL CIRCLE SHOULD BE DRAWN WITH CHALK OR CARBON, HOLDING IT IN THE RIGHT HAND WHILE THE FIST OF THE LEFT IS TIGHTLY CLOSED WITH THE THUMB COVERING AND PRESSING THE INDEX AND MIDDLE FINGERS, (DRAWING SHO-ULD BE MADE FROM LEFT TO RIGHT, FOLLO-WING THE MOVEMENT OF THE SUN) AROUND THE CIRCLE SHOULD BE INCRIBED NAME OR NAMES AND WORDS OF PROTECTION, ACCOR-DING TO THE NATURE OF THE RITUAL, BUT THE INSCRIBING SHOULD BE DONE WITH THOUGHT, FEELING AND WILLING, PUTTING THE INTEN-TION INTO THE WRITING OF WORDS.

" YAT-HA-AH-HU-VAI-RIO " ∴ ꝇꝍ ꝏ꞉ ꝏ ꝏꝏꝏ ꝏ꞉ ꝏꝏꝏ ꞉ ꝏꝏꝏ ∴ IS MASTER PROTECTION, " THE WILL OF THE LORD IS THE LAW OF RIGHT-EUSNESS.-" - OR. YAT-HA-AM-HU-VO. ꞉ꝏꝏꝏ꞉ꝏ꞉ꝏꝏꝏ꞉ꝏ꞉ꝏꝏ꞉ THE WILL OF THE LORD IS MIGHT.

REMEMBER THAT THE MAGICAL CIRCLE IS
PROTECTION FROM YOUR OWN VOLITIONAL
AND INTENTIONAL EMANATIONS, WHICH
GROW TO THE EXTENT OF BEING VERY
DANGEROUS WHEN THEY TRY TO TAKE
POSSESION OF YOUR BODY AND MIND,

PROJECTION VIEW FROM ABOVE.

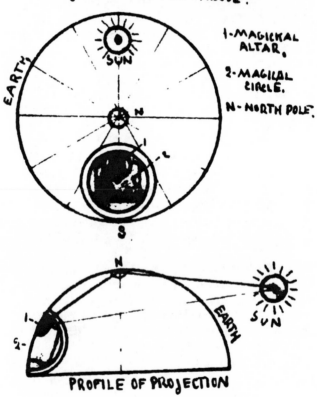

1- MAGICKAL
   ALTAR.

2- MAGICAL
   CIRCLE.

N- NORTH POLE.

PROFILE OF PROJECTION

MAGICAL CIRCLE.. AND THE ALTAR.

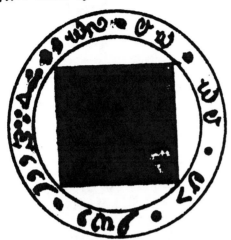

THE MAGICAL WAND IS TO BE MADE FROM WOOD
HOLLOWED INSIDE WITH MAGNETISED STEEL WIRE
INSERTED SO THAT THE HANDHOLDS PART WITH
THE NORTH POLE WHILE THE SOUTH POLE IS AT THE
END, WITH A CRYSTAL OF TOURMALINE ATTACH
ED TO IT. (LENGHT OF MAGICAL WANDT, ARM,
OR POREARM.).

N ━━━━━━━━━━━━━━━━━━━━━━━━ S

COPPER WIRE THEN IS WOUND AROUND THE WAND IN A
RIGHT HANDED SPIRAL TERMINATING IN A COPPER
PLATE HELPING TO HOLD THE TOURMALINE.

ALTAR REPRESENTS THE FIELD ON WHICH THE ACTUAL
WORK WILL BE DONE IN SCALE.

SENDING THE LOADED WITH FEELINGS AND WILLI-
FIED THOUGHT IS THE WORK OF MAGICK. IF IT IS
DONE CORRECTLY, IT IS HARMONIOUS WITH THE
OTHER POWERS, AND WHEN SENT ACCORDING
TO THE MAGNETIC POLE AND ELECTRIC SUN, IT
WILL ATTRACT THE POWERS OF SAME VIBRATIONS

GROWING IN STRENGHT UNTOLD NUMBER OF
TIMES, AND OBEDIENT TO THE CONSCIOUS THOUGHT
WHICH CALLED THE POWERS IN HARMONIOUS
UNIT. THIS PROCESS IS THE INWOKING OF
HEAVENLY HOST.

REMEMBER THO CONSCIOUS WILLIFIED AND
FILLED WITH FEELINGS THOUGHT IS THE LEA-
DER. YOUR THOUGHT, AND THEREFORE YOU
MUST BE PROTECTED, AND ALSO STRONG
ENOUGH TO WITSTAND AND WITHOLD A POS-
SIBLE REBOUND.

INWOCATION IS CENTERING THE THOUGHT
ON ONE POINT, ENDOWING IT WITH FEELINGS
AND ARMING IT WITH WILL, THEN TROUGH
MAGNETIC, ELECTRIC POWER ADHERENT
TO IT, THE THOUGHT BECOMES CRYSTALLO-
GRAPHIC AXIS, AROUND WHICH THE POWERS
CENTER, UPBUILD IT AND MATERIALISE
BECOMING MANIFEST.

WORKING ACCORDING TO THE NORTH
POLE AND THE SUN, THE THOUGHT BE-
COMES THE LEVER WORKING OUT THINGS
IN SCALE ■ IN HARMONY WITH THE SACRED
FORMULA — "AS ABOVE - SO BELOW, AS BELOW
SO ABOVE ".

FOR INWOKING THE ELEMENTAL, AWAKEN
THE SPIRIT ESSENCE OF IT IN YOU, AND
PROJECT IT IN THE SPACE OUTLINED FOR
IT OUTSIDE THE MAGICAL CIRCLE.
THE WISH, DESIRE AND WILL OF HIE-
ROPHANT IS THE AXIS AROUND WHICH
THRU THE ATTRACTION OF THE HARMO-
NIOUS POWERS THE IMAGE OF ENTITY
OF INVOKED ELEMENTAL OR SPIRIT

126

IS MANIFESTED . "LIKE ATTRACTS ALIKE"

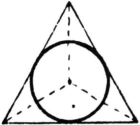

POINT OF CONCEN-
TRATIVE PROJEC-
TION.

FORM OF SPACE FOR ELEMENTAL TO APPEAR.
MADE OUTSIDE OF THE MAGICAL CIRCLE.
RITUAL , CEREMONIAL , CANDLES , IN

CPSIA information can be obtained at www.ICGtesting.com
Printed in the USA
LVOW06s1723110514

385316LV00002B/454/P